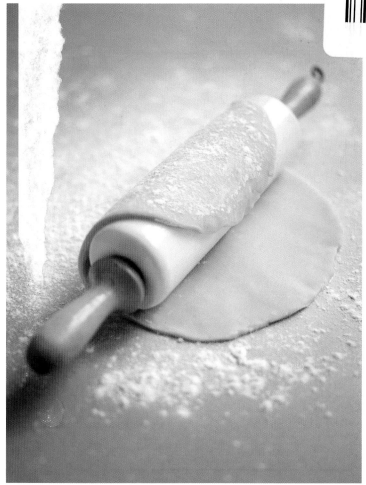

Allergy-free
COOKBOOK

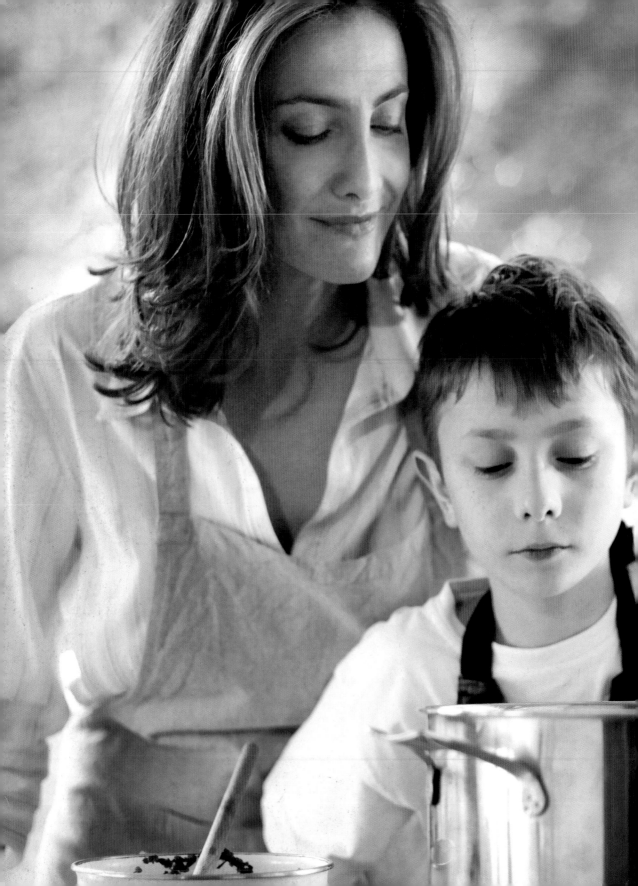

Allergy-free
COOKBOOK

Alice Sherwood

LONDON, NEW YORK, MELBOURNE, MUNICH, DELHI

Project editor Helen Murray
Senior editor Esther Ripley
Project designer Vicky Read
Senior art editor Anne Fisher
DTP designer Sonia Charbonnier
Jacket designer Nicola Powling
Production controller Luca Frassinetti
Managing editor Penny Warren
Managing art editor Marianne Markham
Creative publisher Mary-Clare Jerram
Art director Peter Luff
Medical advisor Adam Fox
Food styling Sarah Tildesley
Home economist Carolyn Humphries
Photographer Kate Whitaker
Photography art direction Luis Peral

First published in Great Britain in 2007
This edition first published in 2010
by Dorling Kindersley Limited
80 Strand, London WC2R 0RL
Penguin Group (UK)

Copyright © 2007, 2010 Dorling Kindersley Limited
Text copyright © 2007, 2010 Alice Sherwood

2 4 6 8 10 9 7 5 3 1

A CIP catalogue record for this book is available from the British Library

ISBN: 978-1-4053-4580-4

Printed and bound by Star Standard, Singapore

Discover more at
www.dk.com

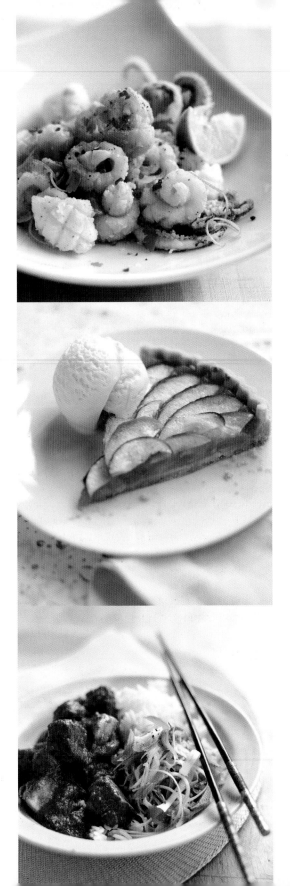

Once a medical curiosity, food allergy has increased dramatically over the past 30 years, even being referred to as an epidemic. When I make a diagnosis of food allergy, I have become increasingly aware that this has implications not just for the patient attending my clinic but also for their extended family and friends, both present and future. With so much of our lives revolving around food, the impact of needing to avoid just a single food can be huge. Invitations to dinner parties and social gatherings become a source of embarrassment and anxiety rather than enjoyment. A simple trip to the supermarket can become a lengthy series of food label examinations and a family trip abroad, if even considered, a delicate military operation.

Some families respond to the allergy of one of its members by severely restricting the foods that the whole family eats. This fear of contact with certain foods leads to a reliance on a small group of bland ingredients. As a result, the family's diet may be safe but also very boring and repetitive, not to mention resented by those who do not actually have an allergy themselves. Other families try to limit only the diet of the affected person but this can lead to feelings of isolation at mealtimes as well as the extra effort of trying to provide two different meals for one sitting.

Alice Sherwood has taken an altogether more positive approach. Instead of focusing on restrictions, she has found ways to sidestep them in her own favourite dishes, as well as exploring the cuisine of other cultures. Her imaginative approach to replacing common allergenic ingredients has paid dividends – a collection of recipes that allow the whole family to enjoy delicious food without anybody feeling left out. However, this book is far more than just a collection of recipes. Alice's positive attitude towards the challenges faced by a family with a food allergic child reveal an insight that could only be offered by someone with first-hand experience. You have probably picked up this book with the hope of finding some inspiration for the kitchen. You will certainly find that here – as well as a lot more besides.

Bon appétit

Adam Fox

Dr Adam Fox
MA(Hons), MSc, MB, BS, MRCPCH
Consultant Paediatric Allergist
Guy's and St Thomas' Hospitals NHS Foundation Trust, London
Health Advisor to Allergy UK

The recipes

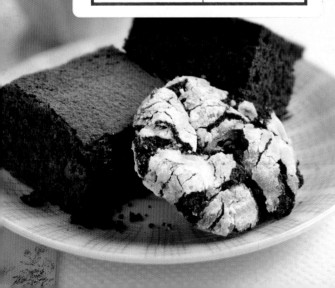

Contents

Introduction

There are many reasons for writing a cookery book. Mine are love of good food and cooking and a desire to share the food I love with friends and family. My very important extra reason is that I wanted to produce a fantastic cookery book that would also work for people who can't eat certain foods because I have a child who is allergic to two foods: eggs and nuts. Later, as it turned out, I found quite a few friends were avoiding dairy and wheat, but Archie's allergies were the starting point.

I was also spurred on to write *The Allergy-free Cookbook* for the simplest and most classic of reasons: it is the book that I couldn't find when I needed it. I was looking for a cookbook that was as full of beautiful, mouth-watering recipes and enticing pictures as any of the glossy books already on my bookshelf. I wanted one that empathized with people with food hypersensitivities and the difficulties they encounter, whilst not treating them as marginal medical cases or cranks. There should be dishes, I felt, that people could eat together without even realizing they were dairy free or gluten free.

"Dining with one's friends and beloved family is certainly one of life's primal and most innocent delights, one that is both soul-satisfying and eternal", writes Julia Child. I wanted an allergy friendly cookbook that kept that notion at its core. Lastly, I wanted to concentrate on freshly prepared food made of healthy ingredients, using the vegetables from my garden as well as the haul from my local supermarket.

Our world turned upside down

My own path to understanding how allergy and intolerance affect your life and what you can do to make the best of living with them, is similar to many. My elder son Archie was diagnosed as allergic to eggs, nuts, and peanuts, although his younger brother, Ben, is not. It turned our world upside down. It was frankly scary to accept that normally harmless foods can be lethal to my child. I needed a helping hand to learn to deal with the problems of never being able to go out for a meal or to a party without carrying a packed meal.

Favourite foods were suddenly out of bounds and simple things like eating at other people's houses became a minefield. People, it transpired, were actually scared to invite us around. It took me a long time to find out what I needed to know and how to explain it to other people.

However, as I talked to other people I realized that Archie and I weren't alone. I found friends whose children had just been diagnosed as coeliac; lactose intolerants amongst colleagues at work and parents at the school gates; neighbours'

Dining with friends and beloved family is certainly one of life's primal and most innocent delights…

children who couldn't touch nuts or peanuts; and adults who had given up dairy or wheat for a variety of health, diet, and lifestyle reasons. We shared experiences and found similar problems, not least the difficulty of explaining to other people what the problems are and how to ask them for help.

Eat everything you can

As I began to plan and develop my recipes I became increasingly wary of the "one size fits all" allergen-free concoctions (recipes that are simultaneously gluten free, dairy free, egg free,

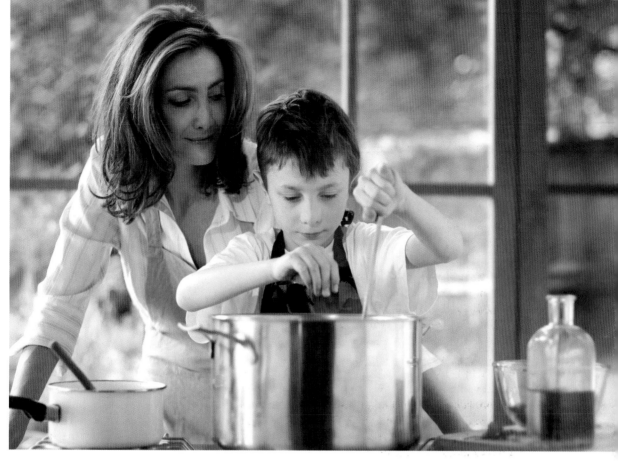

▲ Alice passes on tips and techniques for allergy-safe cooking to her nine-year-old son, Archie.

and nut free, and quite often sesame, soya, fish, and seafood free, too) that I found in most allergy cookbooks. I couldn't see why not being able to eat one or two things meant having no choice about the rest. My philosophy is – why avoid all those things if you don't need to? You will be missing out – not just on taste and enjoyment but quite possibly on nutrients, too. The health implications of that worried me, especially for anyone feeding children.

Four big food problems

Most countries have a list of 10 to 14 possible allergens in food for labelling purposes but of these there are four major allergens (the "Big Four") that cause huge problems for sufferers and for anyone who cooks for them; these are gluten (found in some grains), dairy, egg, and nuts. Research shows that most people with problems are actually allergic to only one or two

foods, so it made sense to develop alternative versions to cater for each major food allergen for each of the recipes in the book. The premise, and indeed the promise, of this book is that every recipe has individually a gluten-free, a dairy-free, an egg-free, and a nut-free version, which means some recipes may have up to three versions, though some need only one. Think of it as getting three or four cookbooks for the price of one!

Obviously avoid fish or seafood recipes if that's your issue but I didn't want to leave them out of the book as they are delicious, nutritious, and add variety. Sesame seeds are sprinkled on a few dishes but easy to omit or replace. Soya appears only as a dairy substitute or as soy sauce. If soya is your allergy, you'll know that the problem is not the loss of a major nutrient or cooking ingredient, which soya isn't, but the way that it has crept into so many processed foods as an unlikely and quite often unnecessary component.

People with multiple allergies find life especially difficult and although this book cannot cater comprehensively for them, there are recipes that they will find immediately usable and others that can be adapted easily. Over a quarter of the recipes are free of all of the "Big Four"; three-quarters are egg and nut free; and a fair proportion of these are also dairy or gluten free, too. "Watch out for" appears on some recipes to flag up other potential allergens, such as pine nuts, that may need to be omitted or an alternative used. These alerts also highlight hidden pitfalls for people who may not be attuned to the fine details of food sensitivity but want to cook for friends and family who have an allergy or intolerance. They should be encouraged!

to forbidden foods. Some were general – toppings to use instead of nuts and which dairy-free milks taste best in which dishes – but some had to be precise, especially for baking: an egg substitute has to replace the same amount of liquid as one egg, and have a similar binding or raising power, too.

If the versions look different from each other or need a slightly different treatment, I've made a point of telling you. Where something is non-intuitive, like a cake batter that seems too liquid but works triumphantly when cooked, or gluten-free pastry that has a dryish feel that might tempt you to add more water (don't!), I've flagged it up.

To make a chocolate birthday cake for a child who has to turn down treats at every party, and to see his face light up with pleasure, is my greatest triumph

My cooking
We live in London and spend holidays at my husband's family farm in rural mid-Wales but my own culinary influences range from French and Mediterranean to Middle Eastern and Vietnamese. My recipes reflect this and range from pastas, risottos, tagines, and rice paper rolls to *panna cotta*, plum crumble, and *tarte aux pommes*. Some are inspired by my French mother's home cookery, some by the exceptional fresh produce we have in Wales. One of the joys of writing this book has been going deeper into new cuisines and discovering, for example, that many Thai and Japanese dishes are dairy free while Mexican tortillas, chilli, and cornbread are often naturally gluten free.

Authentic food is important to me. Classic recipes can sometimes be improved upon but why muck about with them just for the sake of novelty? Besides which, to make many of the recipes in egg-, dairy-, and gluten-free forms involves nifty substitutions and unfamiliar ingredients, so I've adapted the classics only as much as I need to.

A new kind of cooking calls for a new confidence. I've built up a file of alternatives

Every version of every recipe has been tested by me, by home economist Carolyn Humphries, and also friends and family – people in real homes with dodgy ovens and draughty kitchens.

Celebrating food
This book celebrates food, whether it's fine dining for grown-ups or children's tea parties; home-cooked treats like shepherd's pie or exotica like hand-rolled sushi; decadent creamy desserts, chocolate-lovers' indulgences, or light tangy fruit sorbets. Whatever their food issues, people want to cook and eat wonderful food without any feeling of missing out. To make a chocolate birthday cake for my nut- and egg-allergic child, who has to turn down treats at every party he goes to, and to see his face light up with pleasure, is my greatest triumph.

For me, proving to Archie that a whole world of delicious food is open to him has been one of the most rewarding parts of producing this book. Whether you are using this book for yourself, your children, for friends, or family, I hope you enjoy cooking and eating these recipes as much as I do.

How to use this book

Every recipe in this book has been adapted and tested to create up to four different versions for each of the four major food sensitivities – eggs, gluten, nuts, and dairy. Use the symbols and text at the top of each recipe to guide you to the right version. Some one-size-fits-all recipes are naturally free of all four allergens so if you need a safe dish for guests with mixed allergies and intolerances choose a recipe with all four symbols, such as Honeyed Welsh lamb (p.132) or Coconut sorbet (p.159). Alternatively, adapt a version to make it both dairy and gluten free, for example, by combining the gluten-free and dairy-free substitutions.

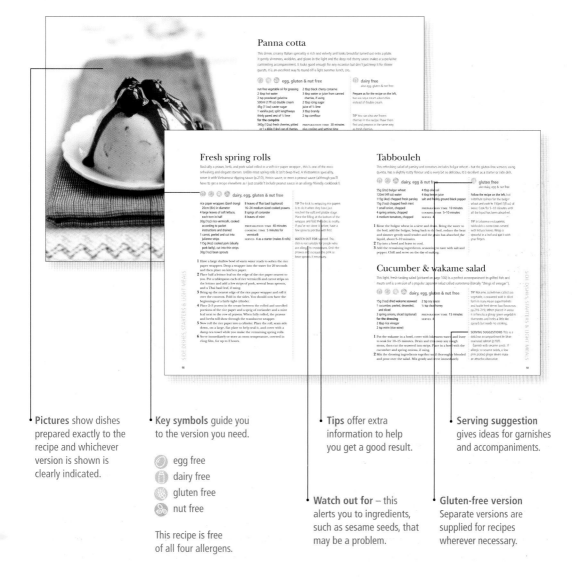

- **Pictures** show dishes prepared exactly to the recipe and whichever version is shown is clearly indicated.

- **Key symbols** guide you to the version you need.

  🥚 egg free
  🥛 dairy free
  🌾 gluten free
  🥜 nut free

  This recipe is free of all four allergens.

- **Tips** offer extra information to help you get a good result.

- **Watch out for** – this alerts you to ingredients, such as sesame seeds, that may be a problem.

- **Serving suggestion** gives ideas for garnishes and accompaniments.

- **Gluten-free version** Separate versions are supplied for recipes wherever necessary.

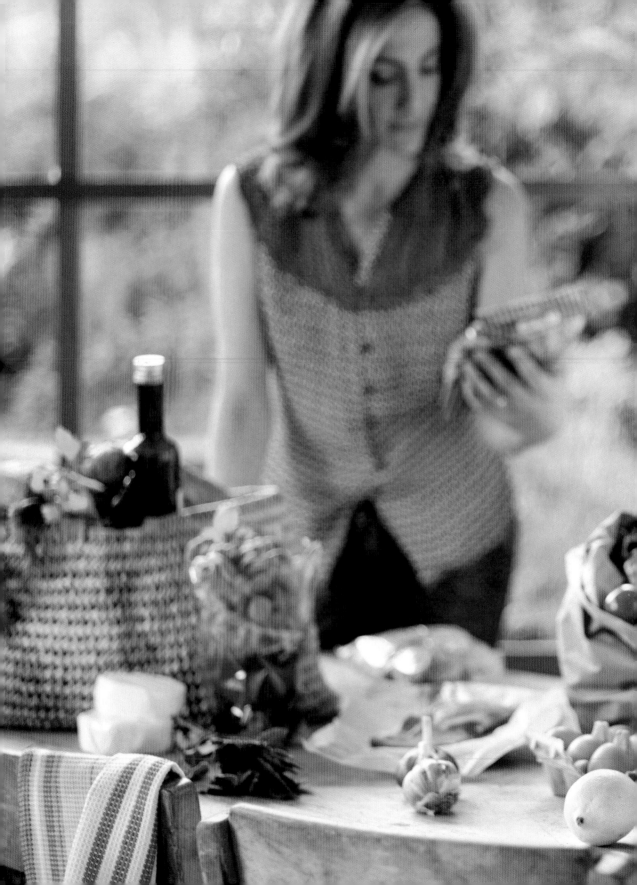

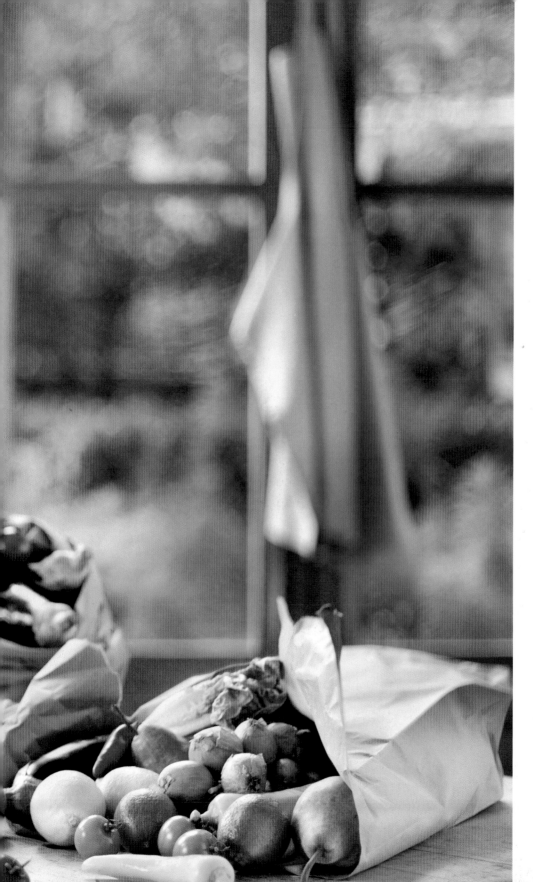

Living with allergies

What are food allergies?

There are many more allergies and food sensitivities around nowadays and almost as many explanations why. Those who regard them as a "disease of modern society" cite factors such as environmental chemicals and pollution. Perversely, better diagnosis has also increased the numbers reported. Some specialists adhere to the theory that improvements in hygiene and medical science have helped to weaken our immune systems. A further explanation is that we've evolved at a different and slower rate than our diets and that we are eating so many new foods that our bodies can no longer cope.

Whatever the causes, allergies and intolerances are now part of our collective experience and although they're not contagious illnesses, they do affect the way people live. You will find multiple sources of information and advice available on them and much of it is confusing, conflicting, and incorrect. My aim here is not to diagnose your allergy or intolerance, which should obviously be carried out by a doctor, but to highlight the essentials to help you to get the best out of using this cookery book. If you don't suffer from a food problem yourself but want to cook for someone who does, what you read here should help you better understand what might be needed.

▼ Party food – olives, caperberries, rice crackers, and root vegetable crisps steer clear of most major food allergens.

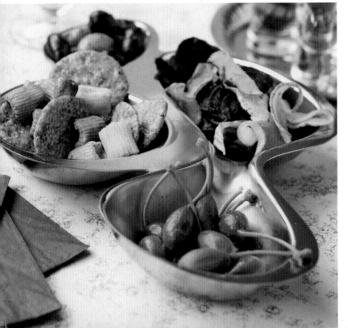

What does it mean?

Rather confusingly people use the words allergy, intolerance, and sensitivity interchangeably, and to refer to many different things. Allergy specialists refer to allergies as "true" or "classical" allergies in contrast to the harder to pinpoint, intolerances and sensitivities. In everyday speech, people use "I'm allergic to it" to mean anything from "it gives me a rash" to "I just don't like it".

Hypersensitivity is an umbrella term used to cover all types of allergy and intolerance but you need to be more precise and clear when you are trying to pinpoint, treat, plan for, or tell someone about a food issue, especially where children and/or a life-threatening risk may be involved. You may have to discuss the problem with many different people from specialists and nurses to family, friends, schools, colleagues, restaurant staff, and hotels. There are some basic distinctions:

• **Classical food allergies** such as those to milk, eggs, and nuts are caused by the immune system. Reactions to them can be immediate as in anaphylaxis (see right) or be delayed, for example eczema may get worse.

• **Food intolerances** are also reactions to foods but they don't involve the immune system and are not so clear-cut in either their symptoms or causes.

• **Coeliac disease** is an auto-immune condition that causes chronic severe symptoms and has a specific diagnosis and treatment.

Classical or "true" allergies

All allergies, including food allergies, are the result of the body's immune system over-reacting to a substance that is normally harmless. The immune system is a complex and sophisticated defence system that protects us from bacteria, viruses, parasites, some chemicals, and sometimes even cancer by identifying harmful proteins (known as antigens) and creating specific defences known as antibodies. Killer cells are produced to destroy invaders and protect the body.

Problems occur when the immune system wrongly interprets an otherwise harmless substance, such as a food, as an allergen, and the body's defences kick in. Histamine is released causing effects that range from troubling to life-threatening.

Reactions and symptoms

Many allergic reactions occur within a few minutes of exposure to the food in question. Reactions include itchy rashes that look a bit like nettle rash and swelling of lips, tongue, face, and throat, which can be dangerous if they block the airway. Abdominal cramps, nausea, and vomiting may occur. The most serious reactions, known as anaphylaxis, are much rarer and are most frequently found in peanut and nut allergy sufferers. They have symptoms that are widespread within the body and occur frighteningly fast.

For an allergic reaction to occur, the body has to have had previous exposure to an allergen: this can be before birth if the food is eaten during pregnancy or after birth through breast milk, or through exposure to food products in the environment. After "sensitization" – the time it takes the body to build up a dislike for the allergen – the first reaction may be from the smallest amount. From then onwards, unless a child grows out of an allergy, there will always be a reaction, but it may vary in strength and severity.

Diagnosis and testing

Classical allergies can be diagnosed using several reliable proven medical tests but as hypersensitivity reactions to food can be caused by a number of things other than allergies, a certain amount of detective work may be needed. Your doctor will also carry out a physical examination, ask about your family's medical history and your own "food history", and may ask you to keep a food and symptom diary for a period of time.

ANAPHYLAXIS

Anaphylaxis is an extreme allergic reaction that is potentially life-threatening. Food triggers differ in adults and children but include: peanuts, tree nuts (such as almonds, walnuts, cashews, and Brazils), sesame, fish, shellfish, dairy products, and eggs. Other causes include wasp or bee stings, natural latex (rubber), penicillin, or any other drug or injection.

Initial signs of anaphylaxis usually start within seconds of contact with the allergen and may include:
- generalized flushing of the skin on face and body
- nettle rash (hives) anywhere on the body
- wheezing, chest tightness, trouble in breathing
- sense of impending doom
- swelling of throat and mouth
- difficulty in swallowing or speaking
- alterations in heart rate
- severe asthma
- abdominal pain, nausea, vomiting, diarrhoea
- sudden feeling of weakness (drop in blood pressure)
- collapse and loss of consciousness
- floppiness, especially in children

Anaphylaxis is always an emergency so if you or someone else is having an attack, dial 999 for emergency help or get someone else to do it for you. If you have anaphylactic reactions, you will always need to be on the lookout for whatever triggers them and carry pre-loaded epinephrine (adrenaline) injection kits. These are used at the first sign of an attack. Even if you then recover, you still need to go to hospital in an ambulance.

▼ An emergency kit for a person at risk of serious allergic reactions may include prescribed medicine, an inhaler, and an epinephrine injection pen. The MedicAlert® bracelet is to be worn at all times.

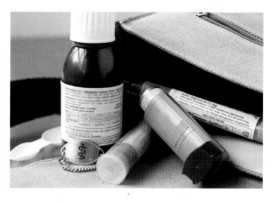

Further specific tests to reach final diagnosis of food allergy and to identify which food(s) and other substances you react to include:

• **A clear history** of your allergic response to food, which can be enough to diagnose an allergy.
• **Skin prick tests,** which can diagnose allergies to foods, pollens, and house dust mites among others. They help establish what you might be allergic to as well as rule out substances.
• **A blood specific IgE (RAST) test,** which involves taking a blood sample for laboratory analysis. The antibodies produced in the blood are measured to establish the likelihood of an allergic reaction. Like most tests it has false positives and negatives.
• **Patch tests** – these involve applying test substances to the skin under adhesive tape, which is left in place for 48 hours. These tests are used to diagnose allergic contact dermatitis (inflammation of the skin) and some delayed allergic reactions to food. They need to be interpreted by an experienced dermatologist or allergist.
• **A food challenge** is occasionally conducted to confirm or diagnose an allergy or to test if someone has grown out of it. The suspected allergen is given to the patient in controlled dosages in hospital under medical supervision.

Because people grow out of some allergies, typically milk and egg, children should be tested regularly to see whether they are still allergic. By age five, about 80 per cent grow out of milk allergies; about 50 per cent out of egg allergies; and about 20 per cent out of peanut allergies.

Tests to be cautious about
Many advertised tests are not scientifically proven and may not be valid. These include any tests, such as hair analysis, that are carried out by post with no doctor present to do a physical examination or take your medical history. Also be wary of cytotoxic blood tests (because the rationale has been questioned and results can be inconsistent), pulse tests, pendulum tests, dowsing, and any tests that measure "energy fields or flows" either by physical or electrical means. Even IgE tests offered on the open market should be avoided as the results need to be interpreted by a clinician. If you take these seriously you run the risk of failing to diagnose an allergy or conversely eliminating whole food groups containing valuable nutrients if falsely diagnosed. This is particularly serious in the case of children, because a balanced diet is essential for healthy growth. No one should cut out whole food groups without medical advice and consultation with a registered dietitian.

Who has food allergies?
Some causes of food sensitivities tend to run in families; this predisposition to allergies is known as "atopy" and sufferers are described as "atopic". If asthma, eczema, hay fever (seasonal rhinitis), or hives (urticaria) run in your family, you are more likely to develop a food allergy, although it is not inevitable. If you have one child with an allergy, get other children in the family checked out too.

At present the only cure for an allergy is to avoid the food you are allergic to, but doctors are investigating ways of preventing allergies in the next generation using, for example, probiotics (the "friendly" bacteria that live in a healthy gut) during pregnancy. Other developments for the future include immunotherapy using "allergy vaccines". Forms of immunotherapy exist for pollen-induced hay fever and bee stings and some non-food allergies but as yet there are no proven, tested desensitization techniques available.

Cross reactions
Cross reactivity means that being allergic to one food can make you more likely to be allergic to another one. Suprisingly, these are not always foods that are closely related. Peanuts, for example, are part of the legume family, which includes black-eyed peas, kidney and lima beans, and soybeans, yet most people who have a peanut allergy are fine with all of these other legumes, but do have a problem with tree nuts. The standard advice is if you are allergic to nuts or peanuts, avoid both.

If you have an allergy and are unsure about what else is unsafe to eat, consult your doctor, dietitian, or allergist, who will use your food history and symptom diary to help them establish which other foods you should watch out for.

Cross reactivity between nuts and seeds is less common; for example, most people who have to avoid nuts can eat sesame seeds (although about 15 per cent cannot). Pine nuts are seeds and tolerated by many people with nut allergies. Similarly cross reactivity between animal products is unusual; people who are allergic to eggs can usually eat chicken – so roasts and stews are unlikely to be out of bounds.

Within the shellfish group, crustaceans (shrimp, crab, and lobster) are most likely to cause a reaction, but allergies to molluscs (clam, oysters, and abalone, for example) are on the increase. Occasionally, people are allergic to both types. It will soon become an EU requirement that molluscs are listed as potential allergens in food labelling (see p.38).

Food intolerances

Often self-diagnosed, food intolerance is a more general and diffuse term. It is used by the medical profession when a person's history and tests show that a particular food or several foods are causing problems but the immune system is not involved or is unlikely to be the major factor that is producing symptoms.

▼ Trouble-free treats can be made without problem ingredients such as eggs, nuts, gluten, or dairy products.

Food intolerances tend to have multiple causes and multiple symptoms. They can be temporary or fluctuate because tolerance levels vary and typically occur after eating a suspect food over a longer period of time and in larger amounts than the trace needed to trigger an allergic response. They do not cause severe anaphylactic reactions.

Intolerances are more difficult to diagnose but should by no means be regarded as a modern myth. Doctors diagnose food intolerance by taking a medical, family, and food history and combining it with selective elimination of various possible causes to arrive at the most likely suspect.

If you have symptoms that disappear when you eliminate a food under medical supervision and which then reappear when the food is reintroduced, that is proof enough of a food intolerance. Common food intolerances include:
• **Lactose intolerance,** which is the inability to tolerate milk and dairy products (see p.19).
• **Food additives** – these are controversial but some that may cause problems include tartrazine (orange food dye) and azo dyes; food flavourings such as monosodium glutamate (MSG) frequently found in Chinese restaurant food; and some sugar substitutes used in low calorie sweeteners, soft drinks, and foods. Preservatives such as sulphites, used to preserve dried fruits, typically apricots, and benzoates and some food antioxidants have

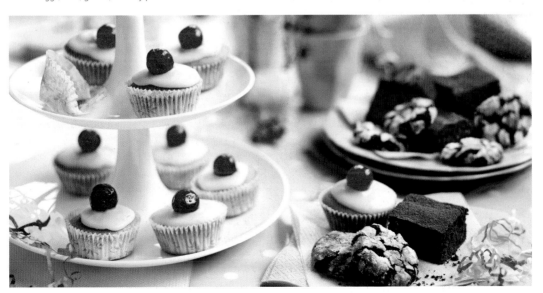

also been implicated. The easiest way to avoid these is to eat freshly prepared food and avoid heavily processed ingredients.

• **Histamines,** found naturally in foods such as cheese, some fish, and alcoholic drinks can cause reactions resembling allergy.

• **Idiopathic food intolerances** is the term used to describe food-related problems with no established mechanism. Foods that trigger them are often those eaten frequently such as milk or wheat. These intolerances are widely reported with symptoms ranging from migraines to diarrhoea, joint pain, and general tiredness.

Every recipe has a version for each of the four major allergens: eggs, dairy, nuts, and gluten

Four major food problems

Among the many allergies and food intolerances only a handful cause problems for considerable numbers of people. These are gluten/wheat, dairy, tree nuts and peanuts, and eggs and these are the focus of my recipe variations. Every recipe has a version for each of these four A-list allergens with some recipes naturally free of all of them.

My B list of allergies and sensitivities would include, soya, fish, and seafood, but these remain in some recipes, albeit with cautions, as many of these foods are staples for A-list sufferers. A balanced diet includes a wide variety of foods – carbohydrate, fat, protein, vitamins, minerals, and dietary fibre. Anyone with serious or multiple food allergies or intolerances needs to be sure they are not missing out on essential nutrients.

Egg allergy

An egg allergy is common in children, although many grow out if it. Egg intolerances are rare. Here are some points to bear in mind when cooking for children and adults with egg allergy:

• **Proteins in both egg yolk and white** can cause reactions. People may be allergic to raw eggs or cooked eggs, or both. Rarely, a person is sensitive to only the white or the yolk.

• **Varying amounts of egg are needed** to trigger a reaction in different people. A severely allergic person at risk of anaphylactic shock will not risk eating even a crumb of a cake; a mildly allergic person may chance a slice, but there is always a risk because reactions can vary in severity.

How to compensate

Eggs contain useful nutrients, most importantly proteins, and are a good source of vitamin D. To replace protein found in eggs, choose from meat, poultry, fish, milk, cheese, soya products, wholegrains, nuts, and seeds. Vitamin D is found in oily fish (salmon, sardines, herring, mackerel, and pilchards) and dairy products.

Tree nuts and peanuts

Peanuts (a legume) and tree nuts (all other "true" nuts including almonds, Brazil, cashew, cobnut, hazelnut, macadamia, pecan, pistachio, walnuts) are often grouped together as cross reactivity between these food groups occurs frequently.

Here are some points to bear in mind when catering for nut and peanut allergies:

• **A person may not be allergic to all nuts** but it is safest to avoid them all. As with other allergies, proteins cause the reaction. Cooking nuts will not reduce the risk of an allergic reaction to them; in fact, roasting peanuts makes the reaction worse.

• **Reactions should never be ignored** even if they are mild, because future reactions may be more severe. A person may have a mild reaction, such as localized tingling, itching, or a rash, to a small or to a significant amount of peanuts or tree nuts. Breathing or swallowing difficulties or fainting calls for immediate medical attention.

• **Some people may react to a tiny trace** of nuts or peanuts, hence "trace" warnings on packaging. For this type of allergy, take no chances with ingredients or cross contamination.

• **Skin contact with nuts or peanuts** may cause rashes and swelling of the lips if someone has a severe nut allergy. Handling the nuts may transfer the allergen to inside the mouth. Even airborne proteins may cause a reaction.

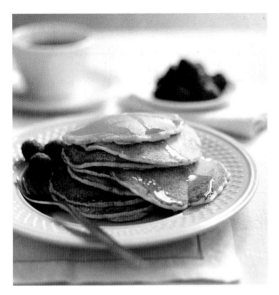

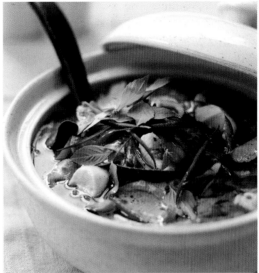

⚠ American pancakes (p.57) has versions free of each allergen and Thai green chicken curry (p.111) is naturally free of them all.

How to compensate

Although nuts are not a diet essential, they are a valuable source of protein for vegetarians. Those with nut allergies should eat protein-rich pulses and legumes, and, if not vegan, eggs, dairy, and cheese.

Dairy sensitivity

There are two main causes of dairy sensitivity: lactose intolerance and milk allergy. It's important to distinguish between them because milk allergy can cause much more severe reactions.

Milk allergy

This problem is frequent in babies but most grow out of it by the age of five years. If you are cooking for children with a milk allergy, you need to be aware of the following:

• **Proteins in milk,** commonly casein and whey, trigger allergic reactions. These proteins are found in cows' and other mammals' milk; sheep and goats' milk are likely to cause similar reactions.

• **Reactions are often mild** and symptoms can affect many parts of the body. They include skin rashes, runny nose, and itchy eyes, gastro-intestinal symptoms such as cramps, diarrhoea, and vomiting, and breathing problems.

• **In mild allergies,** small amounts of processed dairy products such as cheese can be tolerated but not milk, cream, or yogurt.

• **In severe cases of milk allergy,** an anaphylactic reaction can develop within seconds and follow from a minute quantity of milk. All dairy products and traces of products must be avoided. Skin contact and, more rarely, inhaling milk proteins may also cause a reaction.

Lactose intolerance

Most of the populations of South East Asia, Japan, and many people of African origin are lactose intolerant. Their diets are traditonally dairy free and they become intolerant when introduced to dairy.

The condition is much more common than milk allergy and causes milder symptoms and discomfort. It sometimes follows on from a stomach bug, especially in young children, but this type is usually transient.

Here are some points to keep in mind when cooking for people with lactose intolerance:

• **Lactose is a sugar** found naturally in milk from mammals, including cow, sheep, goats, buffalo, and human milk. People who are intolerant of lactose do not produce enough of the enzyme lactase, which breaks milk down in the gut so it can be properly absorbed. This produces symptoms such as bloating, stomach pain, and diarrhoea.

• **The amount of lactose needed** to cause the symptoms may vary with age. Babies are more sensitive; adults with lactose intolerance can sometimes take small quantities of milk without incurring any symptoms.

How to compensate

Dairy foods are a valuable source of protein, fat, carbohydrate, and vitamin D as well as being rich in calcium, which is essential for strong, healthy bones and teeth. If you don't eat dairy foods, choose calcium-enriched soya or other dairy-free milks and include leafy vegetables, wholegrain bread, pulses, dried fruit, nuts and seeds, tinned sardines or salmon, and calcium and vitamin D fortified bread and orange juice in your diet.

Gluten and wheat

Gluten is the cause of coeliac disease, a serious and lifelong auto-immune condition. Other wheat

▼ Delicious dairy-free smoothies (p.59) can be made from a variety of milk and yogurt substitutes.

proteins can cause classical allergies, while intolerances to wheat can be due to multiple and varied causes.

Coeliac disease

Coeliac disease is a serious permanent condition caused by a reaction to gluten in food, which affects up to 1 in 100 people in the UK. The disease is genetic and the risk is increased if other family members are sufferers, but it is not inevitable.

Coeliac is an auto-immune disease, which means the body produces antibodies that attack its own tissues. The villi that line the gut are attacked and damaged, which leads to problems in absorbing essential nutrients in food. Symptoms can be mild, moderate, or serious and include stomach pain, bloating, diarrhoea, and nausea. Although a reaction may follow soon after eating even a little gluten, it does not cause rapid or extreme symptoms, although severely affected sufferers may suffer from violent symptoms known as "coeliac shock".

Because the symptoms can be vague though severe (and can be confused with irritable bowel

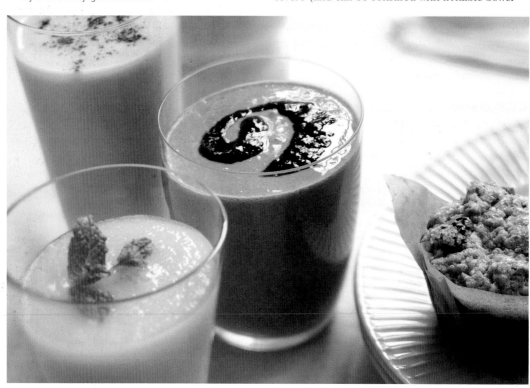

syndrome, wheat intolerance, or symptoms of stress), recognizing and diagnosing the problem can be a drawn out and sometimes distressing process. The problem may go undiagnosed for years leading to long-term complications such as anaemia, weight loss, hair loss, osteoporosis, infertility, joint/bone pain, and malnutrition. The only reliable method of diagnosis is a gut biopsy.

Some useful information when cooking for coeliacs includes the following:
• **Attacks are triggered by gluten,** a protein found in many cereals including wheat, barley, rye, oats, spelt, triticale, and kamut. Products that contain gluten find their way into a great many processed foods, so understanding the composition of foods is essential. A few "borderline" grains, such as oats, may be tolerated.
• **A small amount of gluten may trigger** the return of symptoms that had ceased when gluten was excluded from their diet. Coeliacs therefore need to avoid all grains containing gluten.
• **A child may find it especially hard** to resist temptations like biscuits and cakes so it is important to find safe, gluten-free alternatives to favourite foods. On a positive note, there are many naturally gluten-free grains out there – more than enough to make a gluten-free granola and provide substitutes for everything from pastry flour to couscous.

Wheat allergies
These are relatively rare and are usually occupational as is the case with "bakers' asthma". They are caused by wheat proteins, typically albumin and globulin.
• **If wheat is eaten or even in some cases inhaled,** the allergic reaction can affect skin, stomach, and breathing. Reactions range from mild to very fast life-threatening anaphylactic ones.
• **Severe allergic reactions** can be triggered by a minute quantity of wheat so all wheat-based products must be avoided.

Wheat intolerance
Foods that cause intolerance are often those eaten frequently and regularly, such as wheat. Diagnosis should be carried out by a doctor and confirmed by an elimination diet.

• **Symptoms can be present** most of the time and sufferers feel almost permanently unwell.
• **Many people are able to tolerate** the problem food if it is reintroduced after a suitable break.

How to compensate
If you have coeliac disease or are gluten or wheat intolerant you need to make sure you have enough fibre and iron (usually found in wholegrain bread and cereals) in your diet. Choose from fibre-rich pulses, brown rice and rice bran, and fresh fruit and vegetables. Eating seeds, nuts, and dried fruits is also recommended. Good sources of iron are red meat, oily fish (salmon, sardines, herring, mackerel, and pilchards), shellfish, and offal. Green vegetables are good, too.

Healthy eaters
Finally, I hope this cookbook will be useful to those of you who are simply choosing to eat more healthily. While the most important factors in any diet are that it should be balanced, varied, and tasty, many of you may be cutting down on carbohydrates and fats and eating more wholegrains. As dairy- and gluten-free alternatives often play a part, I hope my recipes inspire you to try new tastes and cookery experiences.

▼ Southern cornbread (p.174), cooked in a skillet and served with Chilli con carne (p.122), is naturally gluten free.

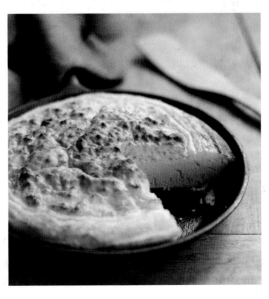

Staying positive

My story is probably similar to yours. When you first discover you or someone very close to you has an allergy you are in a state of shock, even disbelief. You can see that life is going to change but you're not quite sure how, and it takes a while to learn how to cope with it on an emotional and a practical level – this is especially hard if you are dealing with a severe allergy where the need to set plans in place is vital.

Coping with emotions

There's no denying it's very upsetting to be told you or your child is going to have to live with a condition that's going to make life incredibly difficult. Yes, some children do grow out of some allergies, and who knows, one day there may be a cure. But for now you're stuck with it, and you need to allow yourself time to deal with the fact.

There's a grieving stage complete with unexpected cravings for the foods you'll miss. There's the "why me?" stage, which will recur periodically. If you have a close friend to rant to, so much the better, just be sure to make it up to them later. For genuine worries, seek out reliable specialist information and avoid the well-meaning amateurs.

> One of the hardest things is to accept what you can't change, but this is the first step

Don't blame yourself for your or your child's allergy. It's no-one's fault; you're just a victim of genes, environment, and bad luck. Dwelling on things that can't be changed is never a good strategy, especially if they are in the past or beyond your control. Similarly, don't waste time wading through competing theories on the cause of allergies in the press or on the internet; your focus now is on making the best of life.

One of the hardest things is to accept what you cannot change, but this is the first step towards planning a future without certain foods. I guarantee you won't have to miss out on the foods you love, but first you'll need a cool head

to identify all the risky situations you're going to find yourself in. Normal activities, like a meal out, are now a dangerous obstacle course. You'll have to learn to communicate about a topic fraught with emotions and scepticism effectively and respond to enquiries with convincing medical detail – and don't worry, you will. How you communicate is important, too. The key is to explain rather than complain, and that's a lot easier once you've been through the emotional stage.

You will need negotiation skills, too. I've never found it particularly easy to ask for things and would rather walk over hot coals than send wine or food back in a restaurant, but now I can walk into any kitchen, ask to discuss the menu or see the chef, and tell them just what I need.

Getting positive and practical

As always, follow this advice depending on the severity of your allergy or intolerance.

• **First of all,** if you or your child are at risk of a severe reaction to a food (see Anaphylaxis, p.15) put your emergency plans in place. If everyone knows what to do, where the emergency kit is kept, and where to contact you, you've got the worst case scenario covered.

• **Set aside time** to plan for the changes that food hypersensitivities bring with them. It won't be a one-off effort, you'll have to plan for the long term. Prepare yourself and accept your family and friends' offers of help – this is no time to be a hero.

• **Make a detailed list** of all the eating situations you encounter and the risks and temptations involved. This is essential if a lapse will have serious consequences. With anaphylaxis, particularly for a child, there is NO scope at all for a slip-up. Keeping a food diary can help to pinpoint risky situations, for example, eating at other people's houses, travelling, school meals, and restaurants, and help you steer a path through the occasions when you are faced with sceptical relatives and helpful but ill-informed friends.

• **Build a support network.** Find out as much as you can about your condition from books, websites, and allergy organizations (see pp.218–219). Make use of your doctor and hospital clinics. To source specialist foods, visit and talk to supermarkets, health food stores, even pharmacies. Befriend owners and chefs in your local eateries and recruit friends and fellow sufferers so that you can cook and cope together.

• **Ask for what you need.** There will be new situations where you have to ask for information or for different service. Be clear about what you need: a hamburger served without the bun; reassurance that the spoon serving your ice cream has not just been in the one with the nuts in it; to see the label on the packet. People won't volunteer this information – you will have to ask for it.

• **Be realistic** about what you can expect from others. People are basically well intentioned but busy. Catch them at the right time and you'll get a lot more assistance.

• **Never stop checking.** Don't make any assumptions; the chocolate bar you buy regularly because it is nut free may now be produced on a nut-contaminated production line. A restaurant may have a different chef tonight who puts cream in everything. The price of health is eternal vigilance. Take heart, soon it will become second nature.

▼ Egg-free world – Archie is discovering that the simple pleasures of baking don't need to be out of bounds.

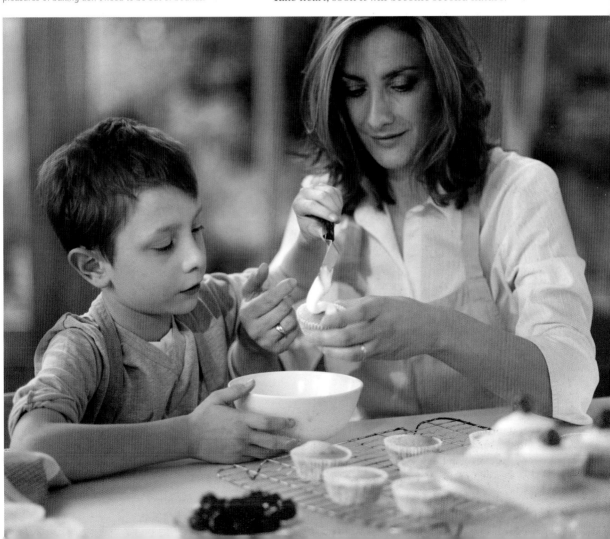

Allergy etiquette

Awareness of allergies and food intolerances is on the increase and the shift in attitudes and behaviour has clearly begun. Not so long ago vegetarianism was regarded by many as a peripheral food fad that didn't need to be catered for. Now, it's hard to think of a place that doesn't offer meat-free options. The number of people who describe themselves as having food sensitivities is even greater than the number who call themselves vegetarian, so we can hope for a new code of good manners that involves thoughtfulness and consideration from both the allergy sufferer and those who cater for them.

If you have the food allergy or intolerance…

Tell other people as much as they need to know about your food sensitivity – and no more. Be clear about what you would like and realistic in your expectations. What you need to tell your child's school or an airline will be different from what your friends or dinner hosts need to know. Give timely information with the right level of detail.

Match your expectations to their expertise. Are you expecting a friend to suddenly become a medical expert or an incredibly gifted and flexible chef? Empathize with their situation and you will save yourself and others a lot of anguish. If you know your host finds it a strain making the simplest meal, eat before you set off to avoid disappointment. Conversely, if you know it would give someone pleasure to cook something special for you, then give them all the information they need and then relax and accept it with a smile.

Thank people effusively when they make an extra effort and tip as much as you are able

If you don't know what's in it, don't eat it. Ask what's in it and keep asking until you have the information you need. If it hasn't got a label, find out what the ingredients are. The more extreme your allergic reaction, the more important this is.

Bring your own food with you. This may seem like the reverse of conventional good manners but in fact it shows consideration. It means that as far as possible you plan to join in with what others are eating, but where you can't you are not putting an extra burden on your hosts. In restaurants, try as far as possible to eat when everyone else is served. If you haven't brought your own cutlery with you and cross contamination is an issue, then it's perfectly in order to ask to wash some utensils or, in extreme circumstances, to use your fingers.

Avoid making a scene. Don't loudly refuse food or adopt an offended tone when offered something you can't eat. Nothing is gained by upsetting people. Just do what generations of guests and children have done before you and leave it on the side of the dish or hide it under your spoon.

Thank people effusively and tip as much as you are able. This is not difficult to do when someone has made the extra effort to accommodate your needs and it encourages good service in the future.

Don't go into the gory details. Who really needs to hear a detailed medical account of your condition except your doctor? Having a food allergy or intolerance doesn't make you more interesting or socially desirable. Similarly…

Avoid militant activism. This may come naturally to those with a campaigning spirit, but your efforts should be directed towards manufacturers, retailers, and organizations, not the waitress, your friends, or anyone who will listen.

If someone else has the food allergy or intolerance…

Always ask for information. Follow the Golden Rules (below) if you are dealing with food hypersensitivities. The person with the allergy or intolerance is the expert on their own condition – especially if they are severely allergic. If it is a child, ask them and confirm with a parent or carer. It may sound obvious but you'd be surprised how many people try to guess even though they may be putting a person's health at risk by doing so. Make sure you ask these questions in advance or discreetly – don't embarrass the person and fellow guests by enquiring loudly or publicly about their food sensitivities.

Take it seriously. Give people the benefit of the doubt. Unless you are a specialist, you are unlikely to be able to assess the condition or what it's like living with it. Food sensitivities range from potentially life-threatening, chronic illnesses to ones with mildly uncomfortable consequences.

THE GOLDEN RULES

- **Find out exactly what** the person is allergic or intolerant to. This must be specific, for example, is it wheat in general or specifically gluten? Egg – cooked or raw? The notes on cross reactivity on page 16 may help.

- **Find out what happens** when the person ingests (eats, or in a very few cases, breathes) the substance. You need to ascertain the speed and severity of the reaction. Are they at risk of an anaphylactic reaction? Are they mildly or severely coeliac? Even if they have a low-risk reaction such as "milk makes me feel bloated and uncomfortable" or "it gives me a rash", it's still something you'd rather not be the cause of.

- **Find out how much** of the substance it takes to cause the reaction. For some people, even the smallest trace of nuts, for example, will be enough to cause anaphylactic shock. Others with a delayed allergic response may react only to larger doses of the food over a longer period of time. Some people with intolerances may allow themselves the occasional indulgence with few or no ill effects.

I'm always surprised when people say something like "In my day we didn't have these new-fangled allergies". I always want to retort "In your day they probably didn't have mobile phones but that doesn't mean they don't exist now".

Put yourself in their place. How would you feel if someone decided not to ask your child for a play date because it's too much of a fuss to cater for her? Or, imagine you are the one child at the birthday party who can't eat the birthday cake.

Celebrate rather than commiserate. This may sound perverse, but negative attention is unhelpful. It keeps the sufferer in their "poor me" phase instead of celebrating all the foods they can eat and the creative culinary solutions they have come up with. It is far better to make factual enquiries and find out what they can eat.

Decide how much effort you are prepared to make to accommodate someone with special dietary needs. With the information you have garnered from following the Golden Rules (see box, left), you can balance your desire to help against the likely amount of extra work and any risks involved. You may decide you want to make a great deal of effort for a relative or close friend, but rather less for a business acquaintance, or that someone with a severe condition is just too scary to cater for – all of which is fine as long as you communicate back to them what you are doing.

Don't promise more than you can deliver. People shouldn't be offended if you suggest that they bring their own food, but they will be upset if you offer to provide for them and then let them down. Respond to enquiries about ingredients, but if you don't know or you're not completely sure, say so. Never guess. My bugbear is the well-intentioned but ill-informed host at children's parties who takes my son by the elbow and says "Darling, I'm sure there's lots of things you can eat here", offers him cake, cookies, and peanut butter sandwiches, all of which have a sporting chance of killing him, and then asks vaguely "Was it dairy or wheat you mustn't have?"

Your allergic child

Finding out they have an allergy is a lot for young children to cope with. It is especially hard for the shyer child as it may set her apart from her friends. Children with allergies are often required to mature more quickly than their peers by learning self-reliance, empowerment, and responsibility at a young age so that they can assess the hazards and go out and enjoy what life has to offer.

Teach the basics

Explain the allergy to your child – the foods to be avoided, the symptoms, treatment, and how to use the emergency kit, if relevant (see p.15).

Tell her not to accept food other than from a small known group of trusted adults, unless she is sure she knows what's in it.

Encourage her to speak up about her allergy whenever it might be important and support her when she does, for example, at other people's houses and at restaurants. She should learn to automatically and confidently ask questions about any food offered such as how it was cooked and the ingredients.

Teach her to always read the ingredients lists and labels on products so that she becomes familiar with the names of problem ingredients and the different terms used for them. She needs to be aware that manufacturing processes, familiar menus, and recipes can change overnight so something that was safe last week may not be now.

Expose her to many different eating occasions – from picnics, barbecues, and fast food outlets to restaurants, weddings, and casual meals at friends' houses so that she becomes more confident about approaching and evaluating the relative risk of new eating situations.

If she has been prescribed epinephrine, make sure she is aware of the nominated adult at school and on school trips who will administer her injector pen. Around the age of 10 or 11, she should learn to use it herself (although she will still need a nominated adult in case of emergency).

School life

Managing your child's allergy while she is at school relies on good teamwork and regular communication between you and the staff. The school and parents should work together to ensure that the child is not stigmatized, is able to join in all school activities and is able to behave in any other way as a "normal" child would.

You should play the key role in assembling the team by fully informing the school, other parents, and children of the allowed foods and foods to be avoided. Supply the school with a management plan (see p.28) to ensure the staff know what to do in an emergency, how to recognize the symptoms of an allergic reaction, and what to do if it happens. Make sure the school nurse and any supply teachers have copies. In most countries, school staff have the duty to safeguard the health of pupils but do not have to administer medicines – although many may volunteer to. Provide the school nurse or nominated staff member with any medicines and equipment, as well as permission to administer them, and arrange training sessions for the staff with you and your child.

Keep allergy-free treats at school so your child can be involved in celebrations

It really helps if teachers take the lead in teaching your child's fellow pupils about her allergy because the most important role for your allergic child's close friends may be to speak up for her. They should avoid food trading but your

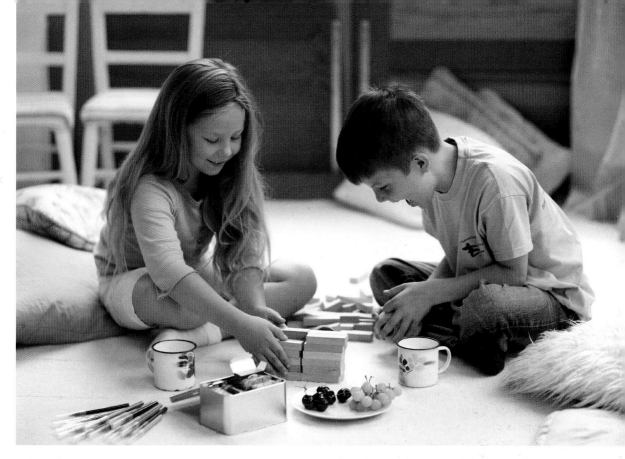

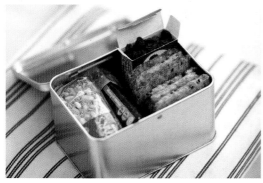

▲ Keeping a box of allergy-safe treats at friends' houses is a good way to ensure your child feels included.

◄ Delicious treat ideas for children who are allergic to gluten include seed bars, raisins, rice cakes, and gluten-free chocolates.

School meals and trips

Decide whether your child should eat school dinners or packed lunches and remember to make special arrangements for school trips or summer camps. School caterers should be aware of food preparation issues as well as the ingredients to be avoided. The caterers need to set up a clear and consistent warning system to notify allergens in school meals and they should receive regular updates from suppliers on changes in ingredients. They should keep the foods together with their labels. Caterers need to be aware of cross contamination risks and introduce procedures to minimize this.

In practice, most schools now ban nuts and peanuts from lunchboxes and in the playground although this is not always observed by parents. If appropriate, suggest a policy of asking parents to ban certain foods from their children's lunchbox.

child still needs to feel included. Involve other parents so that close friends keep a box of allergy-safe treats at their houses for when she visits. This helps your child to feel welcome and relaxed around food. Also, keep allergy-free treats at school so that your child can be involved in birthdays and other celebrations. Arrange with the school that there is a safe food shelf – an area where your child's foods, packed lunches, snacks, and treats, can be stored in a marked and, if necessary, lockable container.

MANAGEMENT PLAN

Before school begins discuss your child's needs with your doctor or allergy specialist and set up a management plan with their help. This needs to be individualized and modified as your child's needs change and should include all the essential information for avoiding and dealing with emergency situations. Arrange for the school to have as many copies as necessary. Here is an example plan.

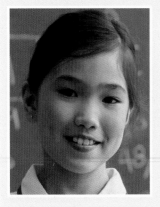

Child's details

Name: Rebecca Lin

Date of Birth: 4 November 1997

Teacher's name: Mrs Cavendish

Emergency contact details: Mary Lin (mother) Home: 01648 42391; Work: 01648 97354; Mob: 07864 34246. Jon Lin (father) Work: 020 4320 500; Mob: 07953 42187.

Allergic to: Nuts and peanuts, raw or cooked, and all foods containing nuts. NONE must be eaten. Any skin contact with nuts or peanuts must be avoided, too. Asthma sufferer.

Emergency procedures

• **Mild symptoms:** Tingling lips/skin rash. Do not ignore — continue to monitor.

• **Recognizing a serious reaction:** This follows immediately after nuts or traces of nuts are eaten: flushing, rash on body, swelling of mouth and throat, difficulty in breathing and swallowing, vomiting and fainting.

• **Treatment – Mild:** Administer 5 puffs of her inhaler and 2 tablespoons of antihistamine.
Serious: If a serious reaction is suspected, administer the first epinephrine injector pen immediately (following the instructions) and call an ambulance. Administer the second epinephrine pen after 5 minutes unless there is a marked improvement.

• **Epinephrine injector pen holder and location:** Mrs Cavendish. Location: Bottom left-hand drawer of Mrs Cavendish's desk in form 5B.

• **Trained staff members:** Mrs Cavendish, Mr Hammond, Miss Collins (school nurse).

• **Emergency calls and what to say:** Dial 999. Tell them Rebecca is allergic to nuts, has eaten some, describe her symptoms and say what medication has been given. An adult is to accompany her in an ambulance to hospital. Further details are available by phoning MedicALert (0207 407 2818) and quoting Rebecca's membership number (GB2939747).

Medication in emergency kit: Salbutamol inhaler (100mg); Piriton liquid (2mg); Junior epinephrine injector pen x 2

Consent & Agreement   M. Lin

Eating out

Although many restaurants are beginning to be aware of food hypersensitivities, when you plan to eat out get as much information as possible ahead of your visit. If you are severely allergic, it's a high-risk strategy to turn up and expect them to give you and your allergy their undivided attention. As always, follow the advice according to the severity of your allergy or intolerance.

Will they be helpful?

A good test of a helpful restaurant is one that is happy for you to bring in any specialist items to eat alongside their food. If there are pitfall ingredients, such as melba toast with the pâté, and you can't eat wheat, ask them if you could bring in a replacement such as gluten-free bread or rice cakes so that you are still able to have their pâté. A good restaurant will be pleased that you are prepared to go to such lengths to enjoy their food.

Make friends and influence people

You don't want to have to explain your condition every time. Befriend the helpful people – at the coffee shop, canteen, supermarket, wherever you find them; it will pay dividends. Our local butcher's shop rang me on holiday to tell me that they'd changed their shepherd's pie topping and that it now included egg. A life-saving call for my son, as it turned out, as I was about to cook one for lunch.

Visit the venue

If you are organizing a celebration, business dinner, or a meal for a group, don't just do it over the phone, arrange a short visit at a quiet time. Don't be reticent: hairdressers are happy to give consultation appointments to prospective customers – there's no reason why restaurants shouldn't do so, too. Explain your needs and any requests to the manager and you will avoid embarrassing encounters during your meal.

Talk to the relevant person

Don't take the waiter's view on how food is prepared and cooked; waiters collect food from the kitchen – they don't make it. Talk to the person who prepares the food and explain what is at stake if they get it wrong. If you have coeliac disease or may have an anaphylactic reaction to a substance, then tell them exactly how serious the consequences can be if you eat even the smallest quantity. However, don't overstate a relatively mild allergy or intolerance; it does a disservice to those who really need to be taken seriously. If buying home-made food from a stall, make sure you talk to the person who cooked it.

Notify in advance

If you need to customize a meal, find out whether the food is freshly made and what packaged ingredients it contains. Ask to see labels on any processed ingredients. Give details of the allergen in question. If they are willing to adapt some of the dishes, discuss the process, ingredients, and risk factors. If you react to extremely small quantities of the allergen, point out that they will not be able to pick out the offending ingredient from already created dishes, as traces of it will remain.

Check for cross contamination

This is as essential at restaurants as much as at home if a trace of the allergen will cause a reaction. Plates, implements, and hands can all transfer traces of foods. Check whether the chef uses his hands to sprinkle nuts or cheese or roll out dough. Barbecues, grills, toasters, and griddles also carry fragments of what was cooked on them before.

Be open minded

Food intolerance is a great excuse to explore and experiment with new cuisines. It will be the silver lining to the cloud if your food sensitivity leads you to new culinary discoveries and dishes that become favourites. On pages 32–35 you can delve into a world of food to explore.

Special occasions

You don't need to give up visiting friends, staying with family, or going to parties, any more than you have to give up good food. But be aware, although your friends want to see you, and really good hosts will stock up favourite foods for you, they won't want to wait on you hand and foot. Be alert to the sensitivities of individuals and occasions as people can take offence if you don't eat their food. Family holidays, Christmas, and Thanksgiving already have their fair share of emotional trigger points and don't need more.

If you don't want your food issues to hijack a special occasion, keep the following points to the fore. As always, use the advice according to the level of your allergy or intolerance.

Always ring ahead and find out as much as you can about the menus and events. Will there be picnics, barbecues, formal events, or tea parties? If it's a wedding, it will probably be catered – ask for the caterer's details and then ring them yourself; the bride will have too much on her mind to worry about your food.

How long will you be there for? If it's just for a meal, a snack ahead of time will see you through. If it's overnight, you'll need breakfast provisions; any longer and you'll need to pack a box, bag, or even a suitcase full of food. If you know the fridge is likely to be full, take a cool bag or an icebox.

Keep your hosts happy by pre-planning the time you'll need to spend in their kitchen and discussing it in advance. If all you need is to unwrap some gluten-free bread or stash your soya milk in the fridge, you'll be no trouble. If you want 20 minutes to boil up some pasta or need a safe area for food preparation, prearrange a convenient time and space. Remember to label your food clearly so that others don't eat your food.

Don't endanger your health by eating something you shouldn't just to seem polite. Rediscover those childhood skills and hide food you can't eat under a potato or in your napkin. And be fussy about serving spoons if you think cross contamination is an issue – you're worth it!

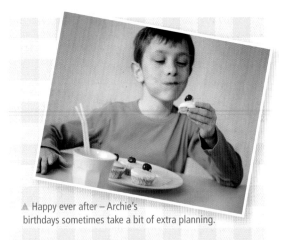

▲ Happy ever after – Archie's birthdays sometimes take a bit of extra planning.

BIRTHDAY SURPRISE

However meticulous your planning, there will always be the unexpected setback. For Archie's 7th birthday party we booked a table for 20 children in a local Chinese restaurant. Hand-drawn invitations had already been sent out when the restaurant changed their mind about our booking – they were not prepared to allow Archie to bring in his own egg- and nut-free version of their egg-fried noodles meal, despite the fact that the 19 other children would be eating their food.

All my appeals for a little flexibility fell on deaf ears and I had to break the news to a baffled and almost tearful little boy. We relocated the party to a friendly pizza parlour and everybody had a wonderful time, and we learned just how valuable an ally a restaurant with a sympathetic manager can be – gradually adding to our list of places where we know people are friendly and helpful. The Chinese restaurant must have learned something about customer service too, as they closed down a year later.

Travelling hopefully

Whether it's a family holiday or travelling on business, if you want a pleasant, productive, calm, and enjoyable trip with no crises or emergencies, it's all in the forward planning and preparation. Airlines, travel companies, and hotels are slowly becoming more helpful and responsive to people with dietary requirements, but don't just assume they can help you; always check first. The responsibilty lies with you to inform everyone as necessary. Once you've done the ground work you can relax and enjoy yourself.

Before you go

Last minute travel may not be an option as most travel companies ask for weeks or even months notice to accommodate special dietary requirements. You also need time to do your research. This is a good time to make use of allergy and coeliac associations (see pp.218–219) as most have travel advice packs, information leaflets, and dietary alert cards (see below). Also contact associations in the country you're travelling to and ask them to recommend allergy-friendly travel companies, hotels, restaurants, and food shops. Find out how much you can buy at your destination and what you need to take. Pack enough safe food to get you to your destination and include some allowance for delays.

Make a checklist with two headings – "what" and "who". The "what" are the essentials you mustn't forget to take with you on your trip. These may include: medical and travel insurance; safe snacks for the journey; MedicAlert® bracelets; emergency kits; and dietary alert cards. The "who" is the person responsible for bringing them.

Dietary alert cards

These are a godsend if you are not fluent in the language of the country you are travelling to. Either make the cards yourself or get them from allergy or coeliac organizations. The cards explain the risks and requirements of your condition, as well as what you can eat, in the local language, establishing you as a genuine medical case rather than a faddy eater. They take the stress out of food ordering because important details are unlikely to get lost in translation between you and the waiter and the waiter and the chef.

Travel tips

Include essentials in your cabin baggage and carry any medication or equipment with you at all times. If you use an epinephrine injector pen, take spares in case you use the first pack. Store them in their original containers, with instructions on how to take them and obtain refills. This also helps custom officials as it establishes them as bona fide medicines.

If you are under medical supervision, get the details of a specialist at the nearest hospital to the place you are travelling to. Bring details of your condition with you in the local language.

In a train you're trapped for the duration of the journey, so take your own supplies. On coach and car journeys don't assume the roadside stops will sell "safe" foods. Take soup and sandwiches to eat on the move, or stop for a picnic.

Most national airlines, given notice, will offer gluten-free meals, non-lactose meals, and vegan meals, which are free of any animal products so are essentially meat, dairy, and egg free. You could also request a fresh fruit platter. However, any slip-up on a long haul flight could leave you hungry so bring some safe food of your own as well. If you have a severe food allergy, take no risks and eat only food that you have prepared yourself.

Peanut products are no longer served on many airlines but there is always the risk that passengers may bring their own. Some airlines will announce that they have a severely allergic person on board, and ask passengers to leave peanuts in their bags.

Worldwide cuisine

When you have to cut out food, it's all too easy to focus on what you can't eat, yet broadening food horizons is a good antidote to allergies. If you don't limit yourself to one cuisine, a whole world of possibilities opens up. Travel throws up plenty of oportunities to sample a different cuisine but you may prefer to try out new dishes in restaurants at home first, or cook them yourself. Don't rule out any cuisine even if it appears to be unsuitable. Italy may be the home of wheat-based pasta but for carbohydrate-loving gluten-avoiders there are also deliciously satisfying risottos, polenta, and potato gnocchi.

Being the product of many countries myself, there is no national bias to the culinary regions chosen in this book. I picked popular cuisines as well as great culinary traditions and grouped together those with advantages for a particular allergy group – for example, Chinese and South East Asian, which are great for dairy-avoiders. Popular restaurant dining choices such as Mexican (Tex-Mex), Indian, Thai, Middle Eastern, and Japanese were all given a place too. With unlimited space I'd sing the praises of many more so let this simply be the start of your culinary explorations.

I've described dishes in this section according to what they ought to or most usually contain, but there are always regional variations and no accounting for the additions cooks and companies may make to classic recipes. The severity of your allergy will determine how, when, and where you can experiment. Cross contamination with peanuts/nuts, gluten, and for severe allergics, dairy and egg are an issue in most restaurants. If in any doubt, the best place for you to try a new cuisine is in your own kitchen.

Italian

Great gluten-free choices include Polenta (p.81), risottos (see Risotto Milanese, p.144), and potato gnocchi (if flourless). There's no need to miss out on delicious sauces from piquant *arrabiata* to creamy *carbonara* if you take your own gluten-free pasta to restaurants and ask a helpful chef to cook it for you. Make the most of Parmesan, mozzarella, and other delicious cheeses, but watch out for veined dolcelatte and gorgonzola. Finish with ice cream or zabaglione.

If you have to be dairy free, enjoy antipasti from the classic melon and parma ham to grilled vegetables, salami, and most breads. For a main course, choose roasts, pan-fried fish and meat, and stews such as Fegato alla Veneziana (p.116) or Vitello tonnato (p.120). Proper pizza and calzone dough contain oil and water but no dairy; just make sure you pick cheeseless toppings or bring your own dairy-free melting cheeses and ask them to sprinkle them on just before your pizza goes into the oven. Sorbets and granitas are a good dessert choice in restaurants and you can make a dairy-free Panna cotta (p.161) at home.

Egg- and nut-safe first courses include the famous *insalate tricolore* with its colourful Italian flag of avocado, mozzarella, and tomatoes. Dried pastas are mostly egg free but fresh ones are egg-laden. Top pastas with rich gamey sauces of rabbit, wild boar, or luscious tomato, but avoid *carbonara*, which contains egg and bacon. For the many nut-allergics who can tolerate pine nuts, there's the much-loved Pesto (p.211).

Restaurant desserts are tricky if you can't eat egg: ice creams (*gelati*) and custards are out of bounds and even sorbets may have had egg white added. If you don't want to risk it, order *frutti di stagione* (seasonal fruit) and make the sorbets (p.159) at home. Nut avoiders can indulge in most ice cream apart from nut flavours.

Mexican

Gluten avoiders have lots to choose from as Mexican is a corn- and rice- based cuisine. Tortillas (check they are made with *masa harina,* which is corn flour, and that no wheat has crept in) are the basis for *burritos*, *tacos*, *enchiladas*, and *tostadas*, wrapped around delicious fillings of your choice. A good one to try at home is with Chilli con carne (p.122), guacamole, salsas, soured cream, and cheese. Rice (*arroz*) and beans (*frijoles*) are green-light menu items for you.

For dairy-free choices, avoid anything *con queso* (with cheese) or with soured cream. Opt for nachos with creamy guacamole, and salsas made from typical Mexican ingredients: tomatoes, peppers, cucumber, and spices with cumin and fresh coriander. Eggs (*huevos*) in various forms are an option, too, and authentic refried beans are made with lard rather than butter. A real treat is *horchata* – a refreshing drink made of rice and almonds, which looks milky but is dairy free.

Egg-free and nut-free menu choices include; Gazpacho (p.85), taco salads, wraps, Chilli con carne (p.122, and dips and salsas. Mango or guava are the characteristic flavours to round off a meal, typically eaten as paste-like sweets, or try Mango yogurt ice (p.158). Egg-allergics should avoid the vanilla flans and nut-allergics should avoid *mole* stews, which have nuts as a key ingredient.

Japanese

For dairy-avoiders, this is definitely a cuisine to investigate and celebrate. Sushi is an excellent option that works well for most other allergies, too. With a wide range of fillings – vegetable, fish, or seafood – it is surprisingly satisfying to make at home in *temaki* form (see California temaki sushi, p.74). Try clear soups, *miso-* or *dashi*-based with tofu, meat, or vegetables and mains such as *teriyaki* beef, *yakitori* chicken or *donburi* – bowls of rice topped with meat or vegetables.

Gluten-sensitives can also do well with sushi. Make dishes such as Miso marinated salmon (p.101) at home to ensure that soy sauce and miso are gluten-free. Cucumber & wakame salad (p.91) and many vegetable side dishes are safe as long as the soy sauce issue is resolved. When opting for noodle dishes, specify rice noodles or 100 per cent

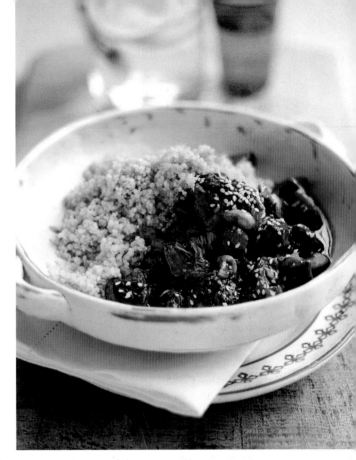

▲ Middle Eastern tagines served with couscous or quinoa.

buckwheat ones. If you like to eat out at Japanese restaurants, why not ask if you can bring your own soy sauce to season otherwise gluten-free safe dishes?

Egg is not much used in Japanese cooking, so many of the above options are safe for egg-allergics. However, watch out for omelette-topped sushi, for *oyako donburi* (chicken and egg), and other egg-topped rice dishes. Make the most of *udon* and *soba* noodle dishes such as Noodles in hot ginger broth (p.142). For something sweet, opt for *mochi*, (sweet sticky rice cakes) or a summer favourite, *kakigori*, made of shaved ice with a variety of sweet syrup flavourings.

Nuts and peanuts are not common ingredients in Japanese food. Nut-free choices include *tempura*, light-as-air batter-fried vegetables and seafood, and *gyoza*, a Japanese ravioli which are steamed or fried (sometimes called pot stickers). A popular choice to finish is Green tea ice cream (p.156).

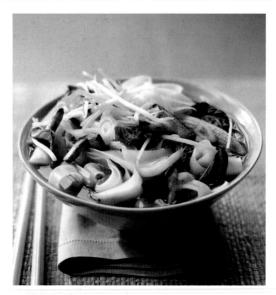

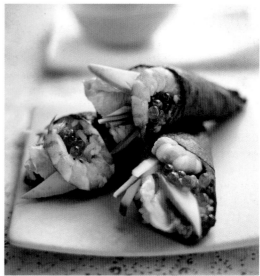

▲ South East Asian dishes are great choices for dairy-avoiders as they are often naturally dairy free.

South East Asian & Chinese

These related cuisines, each with their own flavours and history, share the advantage that they are all virtually dairy free and have rice at the heart of their cooking. The tradition is to share dishes between diners, so make sure you're not sharing spoons or transferring allergens as you do.

Good choices for dairy avoiders include soups, stir fries, many *dim sum*, roast meats, and dipping sauces. Enjoy creamy coconut curries including Thai green chicken curry (p.111), as well as Singapore, Chiang Mai, and other noodle dishes. South East Asian sweet dishes tend to be based on coconut and bean paste rather than dairy.

For gluten-free eating, concentrate on rice. Fresh spring rolls (p.90) combine fresh herbs with pork and prawns; Prawn dumplings (p.103) are another option. Thai and Laotian curries and salads use mostly lime, fish sauce, chillies, and palm sugar for flavouring, but soy sauce is an issue, so cook at home or take your own gluten-free version to restaurants. There are numerous rice-based desserts including Thai sticky rice with coconut and mango.

Egg frequently declares itself as an ingredient in this cuisine in egg noodles (usually non-rice noodles), egg-drop, and other egg-based soups and egg-fried rice. In Vietnamese food, avoid egg pancakes (*trung trang*), prawn mousse on sugarcane, and prawn toasts. Opt for salads, rice noodle dishes (such as Noodles in hot ginger broth, p.142), and stews. The fluffy white Chinese steamed buns called *mantou* use yeast as a raising agent rather than egg. The filled version *baozi* have fillings that are mostly egg free too.

If you are seriously nut or peanut allergic, South East Asian and Chinese food is best made at home because chopped peanuts find their way into everything and use of peanut oil (mostly unrefined) is widespread. For the home cook, try Thai green chicken curry (p.111), Vietnamese beef stew (p.124), and Asian slaw (p.212). In other recipes, replace chopped nuts with sesame seeds or toasted pine nuts, if you are able to eat them. Finish with Coconut sorbet (p.159), served with fresh tropical fruits.

Indian

If you are avoiding gluten, then problem-free Indian meals will be rice based. Most Indian cooks don't use flour as a thickener for curries, using almonds, yogurt or cream, or a vegetable-based

sauce instead. The northern Indian flatbreads will largely be ruled out, but check out split pea *moong dhal* pancakes – a popular snack food, and rice and lentil *dosas*, which are served hot with chutneys. *Dhals*, the bean and pulse dishes that are an Indian staple, are the inspiration for Scallops & prawns with lentils (p.105). The flavours of Indian food are so complex that even if you cannot tolerate chilli, you can omit it and still capture the essence of the cuisine.

Tuck into Indian desserts, such as *kheer*, an almond and cardamom-scented rice pudding, or *kulfi*, a condensed milk, pistachio, and almond ice cream.

For dairy avoiders, grills and kebabs are the safest choices as many curries contain yogurt, *ghee*, or cream. One that doesn't is *vindaloo*. Alternatively, make Indian dishes at home such as Spinach & yogurt lamb curry (p.131) in the dairy-free version. Opt for oven-baked flatbreads such as tandoori *roti* and *chapatti*, and check that fried breads like *poori* and *paratha* have been made using oil rather than *ghee* (clarified butter). Avoid *naan* and breads with yogurt in them. For dessert try dairy-free Mango yogurt ice (p.158).

Eggs tend to be a named feature rather than a hidden ingredient in Indian dishes. So you can enjoy most breads (avoid *naan* which may contain egg), rice, meat and vegetable curries, pickles and chutneys, as well as *lassi*, a cooling yogurt drink.

If you are nut or peanut allergic, beware of the ground almonds and pistachios in many curries, breads, and sweet dishes. In restaurants, check the oil used if ordering fried foods. Kebabs, grilled fish, and tandoori dishes are good choices with Raita (p.213) or make your own Tandoori fish (p.98). Enjoy sweet treats such as *gulab jamun*, fried milk balls in a rose-scented syrup.

French
Gluten-avoiders should steer clear of pastries and pâtisserie in the knowledge that you can make your own Croissants (p.54) and Pains au chocolat (p.66). Many *galettes de sarrasin* (buckwheat pancakes) are made with no added wheat flour,

but check first. Avoid stews, which may be flour thickened, and opt for grills, *steak au poivre*, or fish dishes. Potato dishes are another good choice: gratins (see p.94) as well as *pommes de terre à la lyonnaise* or *boulangère*. Bring your own bread to indulge in fine cheeses, but avoid veined ones such as Roquefort, as they may contain mould cultured from bread. Gluten-free desserts include *îles flottantes* (poached meringues on a vanilla custard) and *crème brûlées*.

Dairy-allergics should avoid the buttery creamy dishes of northern France and opt for the southern cuisine where olive oil is the rule. Choose classic salads like tuna-based *niçoise* and sauce-free grills and steaks (though note *béarnaise* and *hollandaise* contain butter), or casseroles such as *boeuf bourguignon*. Opt for simple fruit-based desserts such as pears in wine or make dairy-free Petits pots au chocolat (p.154) at home.

> Even if you cannot tolerate chilli you can omit it in cooking and still capture the essence of Indian cuisine

Good egg-free choices for starters and mains include onion soup, *coq au vin*, *steak frites*, and *confit de canard*. Avoid sauces, most pastries, and desserts other than simple fruit ones or egg white-free sorbets. At home make egg-free versions of Crêpes (p.162) and Bacon & onion quiche (p.84).

Nuts more than peanuts find their way into many French dishes and hors d'oeuvres often involve nuts. You may be able to choose carefully from baguettes, *pains de campagne*, *pains au chocolat*, *palmiers*, and sweet fruit tarts as they don't usually contain nuts, but if nut traces are an issue avoid them all and make your own French-style bread (p.170), Pain au chocolat (p.65), and Tarte aux pommes (p.149).

Shopping

Strategies for food-sensitive people begin with smart shopping. There is lots of good food that you can eat out there, if you know where to find it. Healthy, well-balanced diets are a must for people with allergies and intolerances, but you shouldn't have to miss out on treats and indulgences either. Different types of retailers have different strengths and they need to be thought about and approached in different ways.

Supermarket chains

Most have head offices with well-staffed customer care departments to answer product and labelling queries. They can send you lists of "safe" foods and those that contain the major allergens, so you can prepare your shopping list well ahead. They have the widest ranges of fresh food and freezer sections and increasingly stock "free from" and "allergy-friendly" ranges. The bigger retailers are more and more health and environment aware and responsive to customers' concerns on these issues, but don't expect one-to-one service once you get there – the person at the checkout won't be able to answer your detailed questions. You may be able to get the information you need at the deli counter or in-store bakery, but don't count on it.

▼ Sourcing fresh ingredients is easy, but stores and mail order companies are also wising up to the needs of allergy-free cooks.

Health food stores & organic grocery stores

The clue is in the name. These are businesses, of course, but even the big chains still have vestiges of the whole-food hippie ethos with which they were founded. This means you can ask detailed questions about the food and have a good chance of getting some helpful answers. It also means that they are unlikely to stare at you if you ask for something a little unusual. They are not always as competitively priced as supermarkets, but they stock a wider range of allergen-free and coeliac-friendly goods. You will find smaller, less well-known brands, some of which were started for or by people with food hypersensitivities just like yours. The staff may have had some health-food training, and if they haven't, they may well have a personal interest – find out which before asking them for advice.

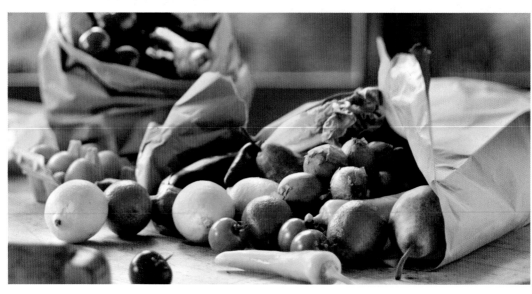

Local convenience stores

These concentrate on speed and ease of shopping. The good ones are friendly and become a real part of the community. They have to focus on core products, big brands, fresh produce, and frequent purchases like bread and milk, but they may well be happy to order in your most regular purchases for you, such as dairy-free soya milk or gluten-free bread. They tend to be very service oriented, as customers are paying a premium for convenience.

Delicatessens

These can be an invaluable source of freshly prepared food and hard-to-find gourmet and speciality foods, but are subject to similar catering hazards such as unlabelled or poorly labelled food and cross contamination described in Eating out (see p.29). For people with mild sensitivities they pose less of a problem than for those at risk of severe reactions. If you take the time to befriend food-loving staff and owners, you may get inspiration and ideas for your cooking and eating.

Specialist food stores

I'm a big fan of food from authentic cultural traditions, as you can see from the recipes in this book. South East Asian and Japanese are useful specialist stores if you can't eat dairy, as there are little, if any, milk products used in their cooking and they are naturally dairy free as a result. Other cuisines, such as Mexican, have rice and corn as staples but not much wheat, and are a useful shopping source for those on gluten-free diets. Specialist stores add variety and spice to life as well as supplying ingredients you can't find in supermarkets, so I recommend them strongly. Many now offer online and mail order purchasing. The downside can be unfamiliar labelling, sometimes in a foreign language, which may not be subject to the same legal requirements that we're used to.

Mail order & online

Ideal for unusual foods and a godsend if you don't live in a city or town or near a health food store or supermarket. The range available online is impressive; from allergy-free ready meals to gluten-free cakes, dairy-free chocolates, cookies, and Christmas puddings, plus all the staples that food sensitive people need to stock up their store cupboards, fridges, and freezers. The benefits of online shopping are that you can research products and compare prices and delivery options from the comfort of your own home – no queues, no baffled staff, and no wasted journeys. You do, however, have to arrange for someone to receive the goods and there may be delivery charges. Some useful sites are given in the Resources section (see pp.218–219), but new ones are emerging all the time. Your allergy or coeliac organization should keep you up to date.

QUESTIONS TO ASK MANUFACTURERS

Food hypersensitivities are now so widespread that companies are addressing the issues and risks involved. Major brands and manufacturers will be able to provide you with literature and a website or helpline, and to answer most, if not all, of the following questions:

- **Who can I contact** about your products with respect to my allergy, food intolerance, or coeliac disease?
- **How do I get hold of** your "free from" list for each allergen and how often is the list updated?
- **What is your company policy** on catering for customers with food sensitivities?
- **How do you notify retailers** and consumers when a product has to be recalled?
- **What is your policy** on allergen labelling? What are you doing to make it clearer and less ambiguous?
- **What is your policy** on "may contain traces" allergen warnings?
- **What advice do you give** to caterers and businesses handling your products on how to avoid cross contamination?
- **Do your manufacturing decisions** take allergy considerations into account?
- **What other foods are made** on the same production line as the product I wish to buy?
- **Do you test foods** to see if they are really what they claim to be, for example, suitable for a dairy-free diet?

Manufacturers & food brands

Manufacturers and food brand companies depend on you to stay in business, so you shouldn't feel shy about asking questions or demanding information about their products and ingredients. They put their addresses on their products and have "contact us" sections on websites because they want to hear from you. They use what they hear to change and develop products to suit shifting consumer needs. Individuals and campaigning organizations can tip the balance towards more and better products for people with food sensitivities. They can help manufacturers to think through the consequences of decisions such as moving production of popular allergen-safe foods to an area with contamination risk. This can be upsetting for allergic or food sensitive children, as it reduces the already limited number of foods available to them.

You can tip the balance towards more and better products for people with food sensitivities

What's on the label?

European Union governments have passed laws obliging manufacturers to declare allergenic ingredients, additives, and substances involved in food processing on their pre-packaged food. Although good labelling of allergens is still very much in its infancy, it is good news for people with allergies, as shopping for food without enough information has sometimes felt like taking your life in your hands! It has reduced the risk but not eliminated it and ultimately, what you eat or give your family or friends to eat remains your responsibility. Progress worth celebrating includes:

Major allergens that account for around 90 per cent of all food-induced allergic reactions have been identified and agreed: there are 14 in EU countries and 8 in the USA and Australia with others pending.

Labels must list major allergens. Requirements vary depending on where you live but most rulings oblige manufacturers to declare the following allergens on product packaging: cereals containing gluten, eggs, peanuts, nuts, milk and dairy products, soya, fish, crustaceans, and shellfish. The EU also requires listing of celery, mustard, sesame seeds, and certain quantities of sulphites.

Any newly identified major potential allergens will be added to the list. A recent addition is lupin. Lupin flour is used in pastries and the seeds eaten as a snack. Most reactions have been in children and also in adults who are allergic to peanuts. Another is molluscs, specifically cuttlefish, squid, abalone, oyster, and snail.

Latex allergy, not yet on the official list, is a growing problem. This allergy to the sap of commercially grown rubber trees causes symptoms that may progress rapidly and unpredictably from skin contact reactions to anaphylaxis on subsequent exposure.

All allergens should be listed irrespective of the quantity in the finished food. Manufacturers must now list all sub-ingredients of a compound ingredient to reduce the problem of hidden or undeclared ingredients. For example, they can no longer list "rusks" as an ingredient without saying that these are made from cereals that contain gluten.

Manufacturers are asked to use plain language and common names for labelling, so for instance ingredients such as *casein*, *whey*, and *lactose* should be declared with a reference to milk in which they are found. Similarly, milk should be referred to as an ingredient in unfamiliar cheeses such as mascarpone, or brands like Quark.

Although manufacturers are required to reduce or eliminate cross contamination with allergens that are not the intentional ingredients of a food, there are no legal controls governing cross contamination in the manufacturing. You may find "may contain nuts" or "manufactured in a factory that also produces nuts" on the label but this information is voluntary.

Packaged food can still be risky. It may be old stock from before the new regulations were in force, or be mislabelled, or have been unpacked to serve loose and become contaminated. It may also have been refined and come into contact with potential allergens during the process. Currently, non-allergenic ingredients derived from an allergen don't have to be declared. If you can refine peanut oil in a way that removes the allergenic proteins, or can produce from wheat glucose a syrup that no longer contains gluten or other wheat proteins, these derivative products don't have to be labelled as allergens.

What I would like to see...

Standardized labelling that is clear, prominent, and unambiguous would be a great start. At the moment, inconsistencies and different terms across food brands and countries are confusing. Studies in America have shown that in some cases fewer than 10 per cent of children with milk allergies were able to correctly identify products containing milk. This is a risky state of affairs.

Plain language on labels. One manufacturer's view of plain language may not be another's and neither may correspond with yours. You may know that Cantal and Parmesan are cheese and that if listed as an ingredient the product must contain dairy – but is it obvious to everyone? It remains essential to teach children with food problems all the possible terms that might be used (see pp.40–42).

Improved procedures to avoid cross contamination in factories and a more considered use of "may contain traces of…" on labels. Nut trace contamination warnings are contentious because the suspicion is that manufacturers are simply covering themselves. Consumers need proper information: if the tiniest trace of a substance can cause a serious reaction, then people need to know that there is a trace risk. The more products without nuts as an ingredient that carry warnings, the less credible the warnings become. Credibility has been shown to be at its lowest amongst nut-allergic teenagers and children – the most at-risk group.

TIPS ON COST

Feeding people with food sensitivities need not be expensive as long as you use a little foresight and planning. Specialist foods such as gluten-free pastas and bread and cake mixes are often obtainable on prescription. Egg-replacer and non-dairy infant formulas are sometimes available through hospitals or pharmacies. Ask your allergy specialist for more information.

- **Various manufacturers**, particularly of gluten-free foods, will send free samples. Contact suppliers directly or via allergy organizations and trade shows.

- **Research supermarket prices** before you buy because some supermarkets hike up the prices. The internet is invaluable for comparing prices.

- **Buy specialist store cupboard staples** in bulk from a wholesaler. Find them via the internet or ask your local health food store for help.

- **Some GPs will prescribe** egg-replacer and gluten-free products if they are a medical necessity.

- **Fresh fruit and vegetables** are likely to form the major part of your diet, but they don't have to be prepackaged in plastic in a supermarket. Check out your local fruit and vegetable shops and market stalls, which often sell bruised and slightly damaged produce for less.

- **Start growing your own food** to guarantee your food is allergen and additive free. Plant window sill herbs or a tomato plant in a pot. Enthusiastic gardeners could share a vegetable plot or allotment.

- **Shop via mail order and the internet**, especially for allergy-friendly foods and free-from ranges. They cut costs by not having shop premises and should pass some savings on to you. (See Resources pp.218–19).

- **Make your own.** Home-made biscuits and treats are invariably cheaper than store-bought and make terrific presents – try making Chocolate truffles (p.207).

What not to eat

The simplest way to be sure of ingredients is to buy fresh foods and cook from scratch but I'm well aware that it isn't always practical. However, as soon as you stray into the aisles of ready-prepared and processed foods, life becomes much more complicated. These alphabetical lists of hazards will alert you to potential pitfalls but it goes without saying that they cannot be exhaustive, as new foods come on to the market all the time. Unless you are severely allergic, you won't need to avoid everything on the list for each allergen. Eat food to your own level of tolerance, and if you do find you can cope with a product that contains traces of your allergen, you should continue to use it.

Gluten

Gluten occurs naturally in an unprocessed state in wheat, barley, rye, oats, spelt, triticale, and kamut.

Ingredients and terms used: bran, bulgur wheat, couscous, durum flour, flour, rusk, semolina, wheat germ, wholewheat, modified starch, or starch. Malt, maltose, malt extract, malt syrup, and malt flour almost always refer to barley and wheat derivatives. Dextrin and maltodextrin can be derived from any starch; in the US, it is usually corn; in Europe, it is commonly barley or wheat.

Foods that may contain gluten
• **Alcohol**: all beers, lager, stout, and ales are made from grain; cider may have barley added to it.
• **Baby food** often contains gluten.
• **Bread and baking**: baking powder, brewer's yeast, bread, and breadcrumbs.
• **Cakes and biscuits and pastries** of all types.
• **Caramel colour** is derived from barley malt.
• **Cereals** (unless specified as gluten free).
• **Cheese**: grated cheese and processed cheeses and spreads may contain flour. Check veined cheeses such as Roquefort, Stilton and dolcelatte.
• **Desserts**: ice creams and frozen yogurts may contain gluten if thickeners have been used. Avoid wafers and cones.
• **Drinks – non alcoholic**: flavoured tea and coffees, barley-flavoured soft drinks, malted drinks.
• **Meats and fish**: burgers, sausages, and other processed meats may contain cereal or rusk. Crabsticks or ocean sticks may contain wheat. Avoid anything breadcrumbed or battered.

• **Nuts** may have flour as a coating.
• **Sauces**: stock cubes, soups, and gravies may contain hydrolysed vegetable protein, usually made of wheat or soya. Some salad dressings contain gluten. Many soya sauces contain wheat.
• **Seasonings and spices**, packet mixes, and mustard may contain flour as thickener, as may white pepper. Avoid malt (barley) vinegar. Distilled vinegars are safe.
• **Snacks**: pretzels, Bombay mix, and scotch eggs; some corn tortillas contain wheat flour.
• **Soups** may contain barley and wheat-based thickeners or pasta, as in minestrone.
• **Sweets and chocolate**: some (including chewing gum) are dusted with flour.
• **Vegetables**: frozen chips may have a flour coating.

Hidden traps: vitamins and supplements may contain gluten.

Things that sound risky but aren't: buckwheat is not wheat and does not contain gluten. Laverbread is Welsh seaweed. Sweetbreads are offal.

Nuts

Many medical experts advise people with peanut allergies to avoid tree nuts and vice versa. Foods containing peanuts are listed separately but if you are allergic to either, read both lists. Nuts include almonds, Brazil, cashew, cobnut, hazelnut, macadamia, pecan, pistachio, and walnuts.

Ingredients and terms used: chipped nuts, flaked nuts, nut butters, nut paste, nut extracts, nut oils, some blended vegetable oils. Marzipan, frangipane, and almond essence/extract are made from almonds; praline is made from hazelnuts. *Prunus* is a term used for nuts in cosmetics.

Foods that may contain tree nuts

- **Alcohol:** liqueurs such as *amaretto.*
- **Baking ingredients:** nut flours, all baking mixes.
- **Beans, peas and lentils, and seeds** may contain nuts as part of a mix or may be processed on the same factory line as nuts.
- **Breads:** speciality breads. flatbreads, *naan* bread. Fresh or in-store bakery breads may be cross contaminated with nuts.
- **Cakes and biscuits:** plain cakes, fruit cakes cheesecakes, tortes, gâteaux, baked breakfast goods such as croissants, cereal bars, biscuits, and cookies (check labels).
- **Cereals:** crunchy nut cereals, mueslis, granolas, some rice cereals, mixed cereals that incorporate fruit and nuts, some instant oat cereals.
- **Cheese:** some contain or are coated in nuts.
- **Desserts:** many contain nuts or have nut toppings sprinkled on them.
- **Drinks:** some milk/yogurt drinks and brands of hot chocolate.
- **Nut oils,** spreads, and butters.
- **Ice creams:** may have nuts added or toppings. Some ice-cream wafers and cones contain nuts.
- **Meat and fish:** check labels on breaded/battered meats and fish, meat pies, some burgers and sausages, salamis, and cold meats.
- **Milk:** some spray dried milk powders and fortified milks.
- **Salads:** mixed salads such as rice and pasta salads, and coleslaws.
- **Sauces:** satay sauce (mainly peanut but other nuts may be used); curry sauces such as *korma.*

As soon as you stray into the aisles of ready-prepared and processed foods, life becomes much more complicated

- **Snacks:** chocolate- and yogurt-covered peanuts and raisins; mixed and salted nuts; Bombay mix.
- **Spreads:** chocolate nut spreads; peanut butter-style nut butters; praline spreads.
- **Sweets and chocolate:** praline and nut chocolates. Many chocolates contain nut traces.
- **Vegetarian food:** nut roasts, cutlets, and burgers. Ready prepared meals may contain nuts.
- **Yogurts:** cereal and nut yogurts.

Things that sound risky but aren't: coconut is a fruit; nutmeg is a seed; soya nuts are dried beans; tiger or chufa nuts are roots – these are usually safe for people with tree nut allergies. Chestnuts and water chestnuts rarely cause allergic reactions. Pine nuts are a seed and often tolerated.

Peanuts

Peanuts in their natural state are also known as ground nuts, earth nuts, and monkey nuts.

Ingredients and terms used: arachis oil is peanut oil found in food but also watch out for it in cosmetics and personal care products. Groundnut oil is most frequently used in food.

Foods that may contain peanuts (see also nut entries)

- **Drinks:** smoothies sometimes have peanut butter added to them.
- **Meats and fish:** Thai, Indonesian, Vietnamese, and Malay dishes often contain peanuts.
- **Nuts:** if you can eat nuts but not peanuts watch out for artificial nuts such as *mandelonas* that are actually reflavoured peanuts.
- **Oils, margarines, and butters:** refined peanut oil is unlikely to cause an allergic reaction. Unrefined oil, commonly used in Chinese food, should be avoided as there is a clear risk. Blended vegetable oils may contain peanut oils. Nut butters are often produced on factory lines that make peanut butter.
- **Seeds** may be packed on the same lines as peanuts.
- **Sauces** such as Satay sauce (South East Asian); *bang bang chicken* (Chinese) contains peanuts.
- **Seasonings:** check any oriental seasoning mixes.
- **Hydrolysed vegetable protein (HVP):** this may be of peanut origin and currently does not have to be disclosed as a source of nuts.

Eggs

All eggs in their natural or unprocessed state and all eggs and egg-derived products.

Ingredients and terms used: egg, egg white (sometimes called *egg albumen*), egg yolk, egg protein. Whole egg, dried egg, or powdered egg includes yolk and white. The terms *ova* and *albumin* mean the product contains egg and are often used in compounds such as *conalbumin* or *ovoglobulin*. *Lecithin* (E322) an emulsifier in many products including chocolate, is made from soya beans or egg yolk but does not cause reactions in people who are allergic to soya or eggs.

Foods that may contain eggs
- **Alcohol**: *advocaat*, *eggnog* and *eierpunsch*.
- **Baby food**.
- **Baking**: mixes for breads, biscuits, doughnuts, muffins, pancakes, pastries, pretzels. Baked goods such as quiches and soufflés and almost all cakes and many biscuits. Bread may be glazed or enriched with egg.
- **Desserts**: custards, ice creams, iced yogurts, parfaits, meringues, puddings, dessert mixes, cream-filled pies. Sorbets may contain egg white.
- **Jams and spreads**: fruit spreads called butters, curds, and (occasionally) cheeses contain egg.
- **Meat, chicken, fish, and seafood** that has been breadcrumbed or battered usually has egg in it. Hamburgers, hot dogs, meatloaf, salami, and fish cakes may use egg for binding. Crabsticks or ocean sticks, may contain egg whites.
- **Pasta**: the dried variety is often egg free. Most fresh pasta, especially ravioli types, contain egg.
- **Sauces and dressings** may be thickened with egg, especially mayonnaise-style dressings, hollandaise, béarnaise, tartare sauce, and Caesar salad dressing.
- **Soups**: broths and bouillons may be clarified with egg white.
- **Sweets and chocolate**: check biscuit-based or glazed sweets, such as nougat, for egg.

Hidden traps: some commercial egg substitutes are designed for weight loss and actually contain egg. Check the label on your egg-replacer. Some vaccines and anaesthetics may contain egg.

Dairy

Dairy includes all cow's milk (whole, skimmed semi-skimmed fresh or UHT), all canned milk, cream, crème fraîche, ice cream, yogurt, fromage frais, Quark, butter, and buttermilk and all cheeses, soft and hard.

Ingredients and terms used: milk powder, milk by-products, dry milk solids, and non-fat dry milk, *casein* or *caseinate*, whey, whey powder, curds, yogurt, yogurt powder, lactose. Check any unfamiliar ingredients with *lact-* in them but note that lactic acid is produced from sugar by bacteria and is not derived from milk.

Foods that may contain dairy products
- **Alcohol**: cream liqueurs.
- **Baby food**.
- **Baking**: cake mixes, cakes, biscuits, snacks, granola and fruit bars, and breakfast goods. Breads may contain milk, dried milk, or dairy products.
- **Drinks**: milky, creamy, yogurt drinks and smoothies; coffees, hot chocolate, and malted drinks.
- **Butter, fats, ghee, and many margarines** contain milk products, as do egg and fat substitutes.
- **Cereals**: some breakfast cereals contain lactose.
- **Desserts**: assume ice creams and yogurts contain dairy unless proved otherwise.
- **Dips and spreads**.
- **Fried foods**: check batter is dairy-free.
- **Jams and spreads**: fruit curds contain butter but fruit cheeses are generally dairy-free jellies.
- **Meats and fish**: some meats and canned tuna contain casein. Dishes with sauces may contain dairy.
- **Sauces and dressings**: creamy sauces, and salad dressings may contain lactose.
- **Soups and soup mixes**.
- **Vegetables, canned or processed**: creamed sweetcorn may have butter; instant mashed potato may contain lactose.
- **Sweets and chocolate**: all milk and white chocolate contains dairy as do many brands of dark chocolate, toffee, and fudge.

Hidden traps: some products such as "non-dairy" coffee whiteners may include ingredients that are derived from milk. Some rice cheese contains *casein*.

So much food to enjoy

Whether you are a passionate or practical cook, there's an extensive range of foods available to you, even if one or more of the "Big Four" allergens have to be avoided. Everything on the greengrocery, fresh fish, and meat counters is on the menu in this book. Make a fuss of a grown up, have fun cooking with children, or just make sweet small indulgences for yourself – you'll find plenty of opportunities in the baking section, which has more than a sprinkling of chocolate recipes.

Vegetable side dishes and salads are such an obvious idea when cooking for people with allergies that I've only allowed myself a few full recipes for them in the book, as I preferred to concentrate on tricky dishes like breads, pies, pastries, and puddings. But there are lots of vegetable ingredients in the recipes as well as in tips and serving suggestions. Pick the best from leafy greens, peppery salads, potatoes for every use and occasion, winter root vegetables and squashes, fragrant herbs and spices, and fresh, dried, and seasonal fruits.

Likewise, if you are not allergic to fish or shellfish the entirety of the fish counter is open to you.

You'll find nostalgic treats like Fish pie (p.96), future classics like Miso marinated salmon (p.101), or barbecue specials such as Marinated Swordfish (p.99). Adapt the recipes to suit whatever your fishmonger has on the slab, whether it's mussels, sardines, anchovies, sole, sea bass, monkfish, mackerel, lobster, or skate.

Meat dishes are often the centrepiece of a meal, so I wanted recipes with staying power– both as common sense cookery and inspirational starting points. Choose from quick dishes such as Lemon thyme grilled chicken (p.109), slow-simmered Ragu Bolognese (p.117) and Moussaka (p.128), and classic roasts for the whole family.

MY FOOD HEROES

Having an allergy or food intolerance doesn't mean doing without. Recipes for breads, pies, puddings, and pastries are made possible in this book by what I call my "food heroes":

- **Dairy-free milks** like soya are now familiar but rice, oat, and nut milks are also healthy and delicious in their own right. Soya cream makes an excellent dairy cream substitute.

- **Dairy-free cheeses** work well in many toppings and sauces.

- **Xanthan gum** acts as a gluten substitute, adding essential springiness to breads, and helping to hold together gluten-free pastry that could otherwise be crumbly and difficult to work with. You only use a little at a time so a pack lasts a long time.

- **Flours made from corn (maize)** have a multitude of uses and have a delicious colour and flavour. Use maize meal for breads and tortillas (p.68); finely ground cornflour to thicken sauces, stews, and gravies.

real problem-solving substitute ingredients that mean crusty, light-textured breads, creamy desserts, sponge cakes, and ice creams are no longer out of bounds. I've listed them here.

- **Ready-made gluten-free flour mixes** are available in many supermarkets. Most are based on rice flour but a mix of flours gives a better balance of flavour, texture, and weight.

- **Potato flour** gets top marks for its binding properties. You can also use it with liquid as an egg substitute in baking.

- **Commercial egg-replacer powders** – use them to adapt cake and quiche recipes.

- **Tofu** – soft, silken, and firm varieties are good in dips and dressings, and replace cooked eggs in recipes.

- **Pine nuts** are my problem-solver for nuts in baking, toppings, and sauces, as are sunflower, sesame, and other seeds.

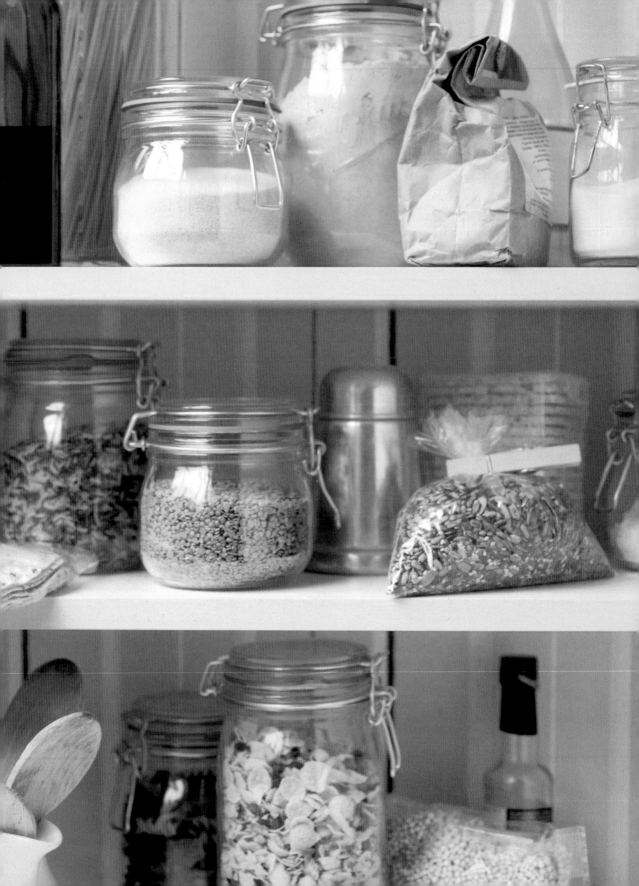

Your store cupboard

Living an allergen-free lifestyle doesn't mean you have to miss out on all the foods you love. Here are some tips to build up your store cupboard to include staples that are safe for you. Use the substitutions table on pages 48–49 to help you with your cooking, and the resources on pages 218–219 for useful stockists.

The gluten-free store cupboard

Here are the essentials you will need for a gluten-free store cupboard. If you are allergic to wheat but not gluten, then you can add back in products that contain gluten or gluten-like proteins, but are not related to wheat, such as oats, rye, and barley.

Breakfast: gluten-free baked breakfast goods, including breads and croissants, are available in normal, long-life, frozen, and part-baked form. Stock up on gluten-free muffin, pancake, and bread mixes and gluten-free cereals such as granola and muesli – or you can buy the ingredients and make your own. If you can tolerate oats, opt for traditional porridge, otherwise millet porridge is an excellent alternative.

Breads and bread flours: gluten-free breads and bread mixes are improving and becoming more widely available all the time. Pick from a wide range, from wraps to hamburger buns and fruit breads. To make your own, stock up on corn, rice, potato, tapioca, soya, and chickpea flours, or buy ready prepared gluten-free flour for bread making. Xanthan gum – a gluten substitute that adds springiness to bread – is essential, as are eggs and yeast.

Biscuits, cakes, and pastry: to bake these you will need gluten-free bicarbonate of soda, baking powder, and lighter flours such as cornflour, rice, and potato flour. Xanthan gum and eggs are vital supplies. Stock up on polenta, almonds, and other nuts – frequent ingredients in home-baked gluten-

◄ Your gluten-free store cupboard essentials:
Top shelf L–R: balsamic vinegar, gluten-free spaghetti, polenta, buckwheat flour, potato flour, white wine vinegar, xanthan gum. **Middle shelf L–R:** corn tortillas, wild rice, lentils, seed mix, corn crispbreads, maize meal. **Bottom shelf L–R:** rice pasta, gluten-free muesli mix, puffed quinoa, gluten-free tamari soy sauce.

free cakes. There are many delicious varieties of gluten-free biscuits and cakes available by post, and a smaller selection in health food stores.

Snacks and treats: corn chips, poppadums, rice cakes and crackers, seed mixes, and potato crisps are good for eating on their own or with cheese or dips.

Pasta, pizza, and ready meals: there is a great choice of dried pasta available made of corn, rice, 100 per cent buckwheat, or chickpea flours. Gluten-free pasta-based ready meals, long-life, or frozen pizza bases and ready-made pizzas are good choices for quick turnaround meals.

Good grains, cereals, and pulses: stock up on staple gluten-free grains; white, brown, and wild rice; corn/polenta; quinoa; buckwheat; and millet. Experiment with less-known grains such as sorghum and red camargue rice. Potatoes and fresh, dried, or canned pulses, beans, and lentils are good sources of carbohydrate and protein.

Sauces, seasonings, and soups: cornflour, arrowroot, and rice flour are good thickeners for sauces. Build up a collection of gluten-free flavourings such as soy, ketchups, spices, and seasonings for all types of cooking, as these are not always readily available. For dressings, have safe non-malt vinegars to hand: wine, rice, and balsamic. Buy gluten-free soups in cans and packets, along with gluten-free stock cubes.

Alcohol and beverages: spirits, wine, cider, and liqueurs based on wines and spirits are usually gluten-free, but check the label to ensure no malt or gluten-containing ingredients have been added. You will need to buy gluten-free beer.

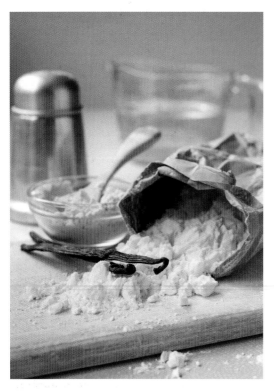

▲ Egg-free food heroes from left to right: commercial egg-replacer, vanilla pods, and potato flour.

The egg-free store cupboard

Simplify cooking and eating by keeping egg-replacers and substitutes for egg-containing ingredients such as mayonnaise on hand. Buy specialist items online or at health food stores.

Baking: stock a good supply of raising agents: egg-replacers, baking powder, bicarbonate of soda, cream of tartar, and dried yeast. Vanilla pods and extract can add "eggy" flavour back in. Oils and condensed milk contribute richness to cakes. Soya and potato flour are useful binding agents.

Desserts: cornflour-based egg-free custards are a great staple, though many fresh brands of custard are egg free too. Keep cornflour or arrowroot to thicken home-made sauces. Packet and canned desserts, such as instant mousses and steamed fruit puddings, are useful. For home-made egg-free "set" desserts you'll need gelatine powder or leaf gelatine.

Savoury: have store-bought egg-free mayonnaise to hand for sandwiches, dips, and salads. Tofu, both firm and silken, adds "eggy" texture to home-made dips, mayonnaise, and cooked dishes.

Pasta: the most useful are the many varieties of egg-free pasta, from basic noodles and spaghetti to more elaborate shapes, multicoloured pasta twists, and lasagne sheets.

Snacks: if the rest of the household regularly snack on egg-containing pastries and cakes, make sure there are a range of snacks such as chocolate, fruit jellies, crisps, and nuts for the egg-avoider to enjoy.

The dairy-free store cupboard

Dairy-free essentials include dairy-free milks, spreads, cream, yogurt, cheese, and ice cream. If you are allergic to cow's milk you may be able to tolerate products made from other animals such as goats and sheep, but they are often just as problematic.

Beverages: the staple is soya milk in myriad varieties: sweetened, flavoured, fortified with vitamins and calcium, long life, or refrigerated. Naturally sweet dairy-free milks include rice milk (good for soy allergics) and tiger nut milk. Buy nut and oat milks for variety. Potato milk is useful in dried form. Dairy-free baby formulas and infant food in jars or frozen form are also available.

Creams, yogurts, and toppings: coconut milk and cream are essential for South East Asian dishes and also a good substitute for milk and cream in many custards and desserts. Use soya cream as a pouring cream for pies and tarts; for thicker toppings stock up on dairy-free custards, almond and other nut-based creams and desserts, as well as silken tofu. Soya yogurts come in fruit flavours – perfect for snacks or breakfast. Buy plain soya yogurt for making creamy salad dressings and dips.

Spreads, fats, and dips: check the labels of margarine as some non-dairy margarines contain milk products. Buy hard vegetable fats for pastry making. Flavourless oils such as corn oil are handy for baking and frying, but for savoury dishes, use olive, seed, and nut oils to compensate for the lost "buttery" taste. Non-dairy dips such as hummus and guacamole, tofu, and nut-based spreads are invaluable snacks and starters.

Cheese: substitutes based on soya, rice, or nuts, are surprisingly good and worth seeking out. Choose from non-dairy cream cheese, Parmesan, mozzarella, herbed cheeses, Monterey Jack, Cheddar-style and those specifically designed to be good melting cheeses. Otherwise, nutritional yeast flakes add "cheesiness" and colour to sauces and Dijon or mustard powder is a useful addition, too.

Ice creams, desserts, and treats: stock your freezer with non-dairy ice creams and desserts. Keep a store of dairy-free chocolate. Dairy-free biscuits, muffins, and long-life cakes are also available.

The nut-free store cupboard

A difficult allergy to live with but less problematic in the home where cross contamination is less of an issue once you have checked labels carefully. If you are allergic to either peanuts or nuts, it is safer to keep your store cupboard nut free.

Dairy-free staples include (clockwise from back left) grated Cheddar-style cheese, whipped soya cream, soya milk, yeast flakes, soya cream cheese, herb tofu, and vegan Parmesan.

Breakfast: stock up on cereals: nut-free cornflakes, puffed rice, wheat-based, and porridge. Source nut-free muesli and granola or make your own. Most basic bread is nut free or nut safe. If you make bread, invest in a breadmaker and fill shelves with flours, seeds, and yeast.

Snacks and spreads: good snacks include dried fruits, fruit bars, flapjacks, and seeds. Keep safe treats such as dried fruits, jelly sweets, chocolates, and biscuits for when others have nut-containing cakes and chocolates. Fruit preserves, yeast spreads, and nut-free chocolate spread can replace nut-based spreads. For pre-dinner nibbles source olives, caperberries, crispbreads, root vegetable and potato crisps, and Japanese rice crackers and cocktail snacks.

Sauces and toppings: include pesto amongst your other pasta sauces if pine nuts are not a problem. Toasted pine nuts are also a good substitute for chopped nuts in sweet, savoury, and baked recipes. Keep a selection of seeds such as sunflower, pumpkin, and poppy seeds for decorative toppings on breads and desserts, and sesame seeds for stir fries and oriental dishes or in place of chopped peanuts. Invest in a small bottle of unblended sesame oil, as a dash adds flavour to salads and other recipes that call for off-limits nut oils.

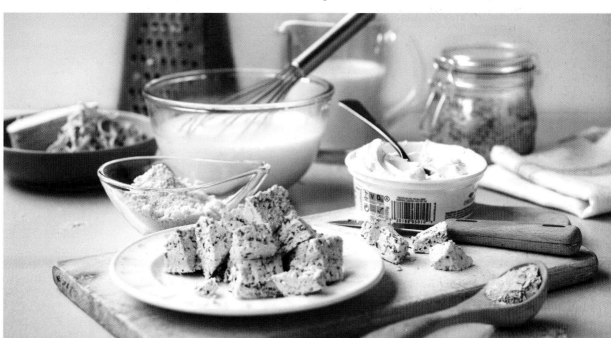

Substituting ingredients

If you're cooking a dish that calls for ingredients you need to avoid, find the problem ingredient in the left-hand column, the substitutes and alternatives in the middle, and any tips on how to use them on the right.

DAIRY	substitutes & alternatives	notes & tips
Milk	Soya milk, rice milk, oat milk, coconut milk or thin coconut cream, nut milks such as almond, cashew, tiger nut milk (chufa), or potato milk.	Substitutes may be thinner or have a noticeable flavour. Some are available in dried form. Fruit juice, purées, and stocks can be used in some recipes.
Butter	For baking: soya, sunflower, olive oils, and vegetable fat-based spreads. For other cooking: oils, animal fats, such as lard, and hard vegetable fats.	Choose according to the taste desired. Some dairy-free spreads contain too much water to be used for baking.
Cheese soft	Soya-based cream cheese.	Textures and spreadability will vary. Soya cream cheese in icing or toppings is softer and runnier than dairy and may need refrigerating.
Cheese hard	Substitutes (sometimes called "cheezes") made of soya, rice, tofu, or nuts. Types include mozzarella, Cheddar, Monterey Jack, Parmesan, herb.	Textures, flavour, and saltiness vary. Melting varieties are useful for pizzas and other toppings.
Cream/ Yogurt	Soya cream, silken, firm and soft tofu, and thick coconut cream. Tofu and other soya-based yogurts.	Soya and coconut cream alternative for savoury dishes. Soya cream alternative with vanilla extract is an excellent pouring cream, or make your own Chantilly topping (p.216). If soya yogurt curdles during cooking, stir in a teaspoon of flour to stabilize.

Note: cross reactivity in dairy is quite high but if cow's milk in particular, rather than dairy in general, is the problem, you may be able to tolerate goat's or sheep's milk, cheeses, and yogurts.

NUT	substitutes & alternatives	notes & tips
Peanuts and tree nuts	Pine nuts or seeds such as sesame, pumpkin, or sunflower. For cakes, crumbles, or curries – grated desiccated coconut (not a nut but a fruit).	Toast pine nuts and seeds to bring out flavour.
Nut-based oils	Vegetable, olive, or seed oils if tolerated.	A mix of flavourless oil and toasted sesame oil makes a tasty alternative to walnut oil in salads.
Toppings with nut or peanuts	Crushed crisps, corn chips, or rice crackers add crunch to a savoury topping. If tolerated, seeds such as sesame, pumpkin, flaxseed, linseed, pine nuts; toasted jumbo oats; or shredded coconut.	Breadcrumbs fried with finely chopped garlic on cooked vegetables or salads. On cold desserts, make a sweet crumble topping (see Plum crumble, p.146) cooked in the oven and then cooled.

Note: if only peanuts are the problem, you may possibly be able to use nuts or vice versa, but many people are allergic to both (see Cross reactions, p.16). Some people with nut allergies, but not all, can tolerate pine nuts and sesame seeds.

GLUTEN	substitutes & alternatives	notes & tips
Flour and baking powder	Ready-made gluten-free flour mixes and baking powder or make your own using rice, maize and corn, potato, buckwheat, chickpea (gram), lentil, soya, or chestnut flours.	Gluten-free dough can be crumbly but don't add more water. Soya, potato, chickpea, and lentil flours have marked flavours. Lighter flours for baking include rice, maize, corn, and tapioca.
Bread, pizzas, tortillas	Various ready-made gluten-free breads, pure corn tortillas, croissants, and pizza bases are available. Check the freezer section, too.	In recipes, use eggs and xanthan gum, if specified, or the bread will lack springiness. Use stale loaves to make gluten-free croûtons and breadcrumbs.
Pasta and noodles	Corn- or rice-based gluten-free pastas are available in many shapes and sizes. Rice noodles or 100 per cent buckwheat noodles are gluten-free too.	In some recipes use other carbohydrate-rich foods such as rice, polenta, potatoes, yams, cassava, sweet potatoes, breadfruit, or pulses.
Flour thickeners	Cornflour, rice flour, arrowroot, sago, and tapioca.	Use 1 tbsp cornflour to thicken 250ml (8½fl oz) liquid. To thicken soups, add cooked rice, cooked cubed potato or bread and blend briefly in a food processor.
Cereals	Rice, corn, quinoa, millet, and buckwheat-based cereals as flakes or in "puffed" form. Millet flakes instead of oats for gluten-free porridge.	Make your own granola (p.52) and then add fruit and nuts to taste.

Note: if wheat rather than gluten is the problem, you can use products made of rye, barley, and oats.

EGG	substitutes & alternatives	notes & tips
For baking	Commercial egg-replacers for either whole egg or egg-white. Or make your own with potato flour and water. Use extra baking powder or yeast and liquid as raising agents in cakes and biscuits that require it.	Egg-replacers may have a drying effect: if so, add 1 tsp oil and also 1 tsp vanilla extract for flavour. To replace an egg, use 1 tsp baking powder, 1 tbsp vinegar, and 1 tbsp of extra liquid; or use 1 tsp yeast in 4 tbsp warm water.
In dressings and dips	Use soft, silken, or firm tofu for eggy texture.	Use bought or home-made egg-free Mayonnaise (see p.210). Use 2–3 tbsp tofu per egg to thicken dips, etc.
For binding or thickening	Potato flour for binding. Wheat flour, rice flour, or cornflour for thickening.	Use flours to thicken cooked sauces or add double cream near to the end of cooking.
For glazing	Milk, cream, or gelatine (for extra shine).	See Chicken pie recipe on page 106 for a gelatine glaze.
In desserts	Cornflour for custards and savoury sauces. Thick whipped cream and/or gelatine in set desserts.	To thicken, use 1 level tbsp cornflour to 250ml milk; add sugar and vanilla for sweet custard sauce. 1 tsp gelatine dissolved in 2 tbsp liquid approximates setting of one egg.
Whole cooked eggs	Use firm tofu cubed and cooked; scallops in fishy dishes with egg, such as Kedgeree (p.67).	For breakfasts, try scrambled tofu and mushrooms. Add butter beans to salad Niçoise instead of egg.

Note: most people who are allergic to hens' eggs are allergic to other birds' eggs, too.

SUBSTITUTING INGREDIENTS

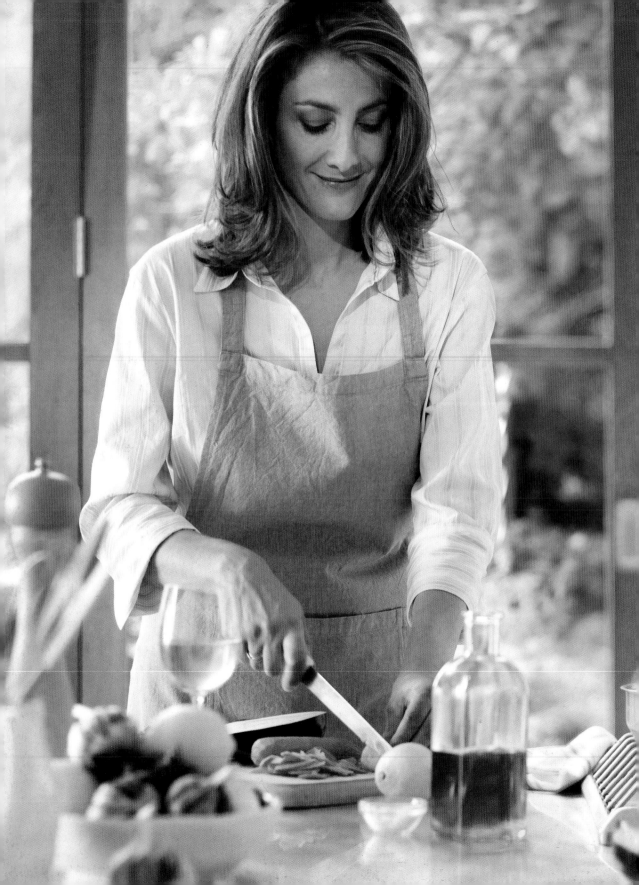

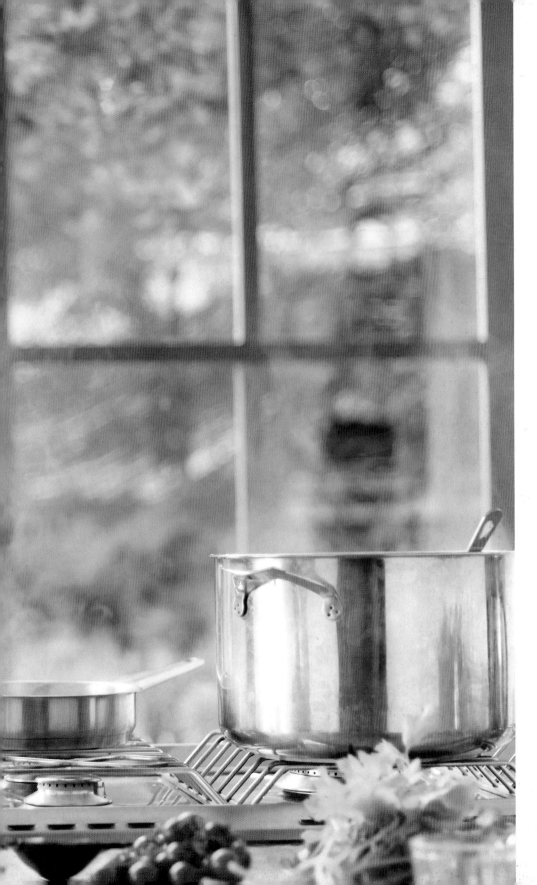

The recipes

Honey granola

A delicious and healthy breakfast cereal, easy and worth making yourself, especially if it's difficult to find packaged versions without gluten or nuts. Make the crunchy honey clusters in advance; then add, according to taste, nuts, other cereals, seeds, dried fruit, fresh fruit, or whatever takes your fancy just before serving. The main ingredients keep well, so it's worth stocking up on your favourite toppings.

  ## nut & egg free

flavourless nut-free oil
85g (3oz) runny honey
170g (6oz) rolled oats
suggested nut-free additions
85g (3oz) sultanas
55g (2oz) chopped dried apricots
45g (1½oz) pumpkin seeds
30g (1oz) pine nuts, toasted
  (optional)
30g (1oz) puffed rice or wheat
55g (2oz) corn flakes
85g (3oz) bran flakes
45g (1½oz) dried apple or
  pineapple pieces

to serve
fresh fruit in season, such as
  raspberries, and bananas
milk or yogurt

PREPARATION TIME 5 minutes
COOKING TIME 10–15 minutes
SERVES 4–6

1 Preheat the oven to 180°C (350°F, gas 4). Oil a large baking sheet.
2 Spoon the honey into a medium-sized bowl. Gently heat the honey if it isn't quite runny enough to mix easily. Add the rolled oats and stir gently to ensure they are evenly coated.
3 Spread the oats thinly onto the oiled baking sheet and toast in the oven for 10–15 minutes or until golden, checking once or twice to ensure that they are not burning.
4 Remove from the oven and leave to cool. Store in an airtight container if preparing in advance.
5 When ready to use, mix the clusters with the other dried ingredients. Add fresh fruit and serve with milk or yogurt.

WATCH OUT FOR pine nuts, which are tolerated by most people with nut allergies, omit if in any doubt.

TIP Vary fresh fruit according to season. Try grated apple with a little ground cinnamon or dried tropical fruits such as pineapple, mango, and papaya.

 ## gluten free
also egg free

Follow the recipe on the left, replacing the rolled oats with rice flakes. For the additional ingredients, substitute buckwheat or millet flakes for the bran flakes, and use puffed rice or rice bran in place of puffed wheat. Add 45g (1½oz) pistachios, 30g (1oz) flaked almonds, and 45g (1½oz) toasted hazelnuts.
Pictured opposite ▶

 ## dairy free
also egg free

Follow the recipe on the left, but choose a dairy-free topping or milk. Try soya milk, rice milks, or tiger nut milk, which doesn't contain nuts. Oat milks are highly recommended if you can tolerate gluten. Similarly, hazelnut or almond milk are great if nuts aren't a problem. Use a combination of the dried ingredients and fruit suggested in the other versions.

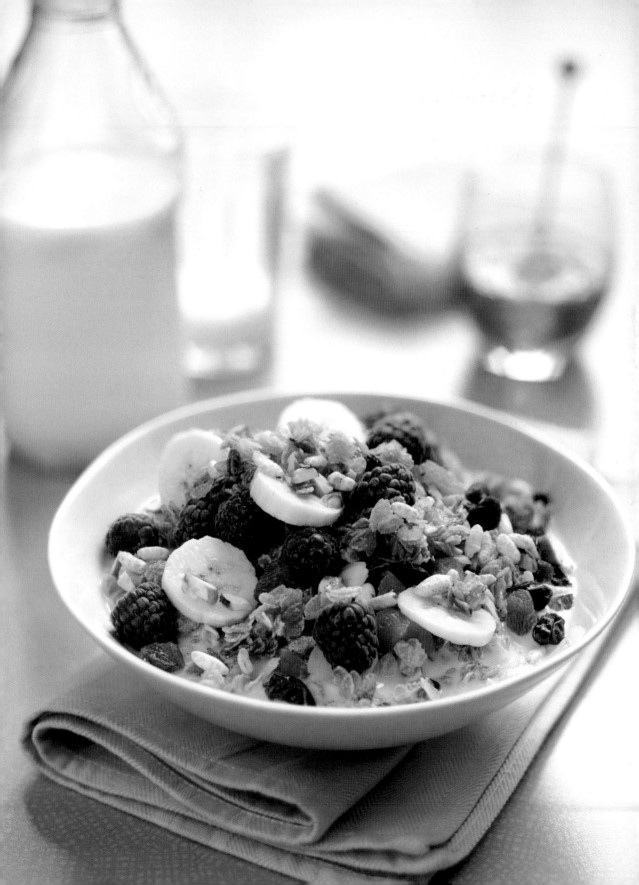

Croissants

The ultimate breakfast food made from the flakiest of pastries, croissants are best made in a cool kitchen with a cool head. Equally delicious served plain, with jam or honey, or filled with ham and just-melted cheese (or dairy-free melting varieties), they take a little time and effort but are worth it – especially if shop-bought ones are out of bounds.

 gluten free

225g (8oz) gluten-free plain white
  flour plus extra for dusting
½ tsp salt
2 tsp caster sugar
2 tsp xanthan gum
1 tbsp fast-action dried yeast
55g (2oz) cold butter, cut into
  1 cm (½in) dice
150ml (5fl oz) milk
1 egg
vegetable oil for greasing

for the glaze
1 egg, beaten
1 tsp icing sugar

PREPARATION TIME 25 minutes
  plus proving time
COOKING TIME 15 minutes
MAKES 6

TIP These don't look as puffy as the wheat-based croissants (see nut-free recipe, right) but they are spongy and buttery, and a tasty breakfast treat.

1 Sift the flour with the salt, sugar, and gum into a food processor. Use the dough attachment. Add the yeast and diced butter.
2 Warm the milk very briefly until just tepid then whisk in the egg. Add to the processor and run the machine for 1 minute to knead to a soft ball.
3 Tip the mixture out onto a lightly floured surface. Roll out to a rectangle. Fold the top third down and the bottom third up over. Give the dough a quarter turn and roll and fold again. Turn, roll, and fold once more.
4 Dust the rolling pin with flour and roll the dough into an oblong about three times as long as it is high and about 5mm (¼in) thick. Trim the edges and cut into 3 equal squares.
5 Cut each square in half to form triangles. Grease a baking sheet.
6 Beat the egg with the icing sugar and brush the triangles. Starting from the long edge, roll up each triangle, curve each roll slightly into a crescent shape then place on the baking sheet. Cover loosely with oiled cling film and leave in a warm place to prove until well risen, about 45 minutes.
7 Meanwhile, preheat the oven to 200°C (400°F, gas 6). Brush the croissants with the remaining glaze. Bake until spongy and golden, about 15 minutes.
8 Best served while still warm or transfer to a wire rack to cool before wrapping and storing.

nut free

225g (8oz) strong plain flour
  plus extra for dusting
3/4 tsp salt
2 tsp caster sugar
2 tsp fast-action dried yeast
85g (3oz) cold butter
105ml (7 tbsp) milk
1 egg, beaten
nut-free oil for greasing

for the glaze
1 egg
1 tsp icing sugar

PREPARATION TIME 30 minutes
  plus chilling and proving time
COOKING TIME 15 minutes
MAKES 8

1 Sift the flour, salt, and sugar into a food processor. Use the dough attachment. Add the yeast.

2 Melt 15g (½oz) of the butter in a saucepan. Remove from the heat and add the milk. The mixture should be just warm, not hot. Whisk in the egg. Add to the flour mixture and run the machine to form an elastic dough. Run the machine for another minute to knead it thoroughly.

3 Transfer the dough to a work surface, dusted with flour. Knead gently until smooth. Dust the rolling pin with a little flour and roll out the dough to a rectangle about 1cm (½in) thick.

4 Dot a third of the remaining butter over the bottom two thirds of the dough. Fold the top plain dough over the centre portion then fold the bottom third up over. Press the edges together with the rolling pin. Give the dough a quarter turn and roll, dot, and fold again. Repeat with the final third of the butter.

5 Wrap the dough in cling film and chill for at least 30 minutes.

6 Unwrap the dough, roll out on a floured surface again to a rectangle, but without adding butter. Fold as before, turn, roll, and fold again.

7 Dusting the rolling pin with flour, roll out to a large square about 5mm (¼in) thick, trim the edges, and cut into 4 equal squares.

8 Cut each square in half to form triangles. Grease a large baking sheet with nut-free oil.

9 Beat the egg with the icing sugar and brush over the triangles. Starting from the long edge, roll up each triangle, curve each into a crescent shape and place on the baking sheet. Brush with the remaining glaze. Cover loosely with oiled cling film and leave in a warm place to prove until doubled in bulk, about 40 minutes.

10 Meanwhile, preheat the oven to 220°C (425°F, gas 7). Bake the croissants until puffy and golden, about 15 minutes.

11 Best served warm. Otherwise, transfer to a wire rack and leave to cool before wrapping and storing.

dairy free
also nut free

Follow the nut-free recipe, but substitute lard or hard white vegetable fat for the butter and dairy-free soya, rice, or oat milk, or water for the cow's milk.

 ## egg free
also nut free

Follow the nut-free recipe, but omit the egg. Add an extra 2–3 tablespoons of milk, if necessary. Use 3 tablespoons of single cream (or soya alternative to single cream) and 1 teaspoon of icing sugar for the glaze instead of the egg yolk, water, and icing sugar.

TIP All four versions can be reheated and they also freeze well.

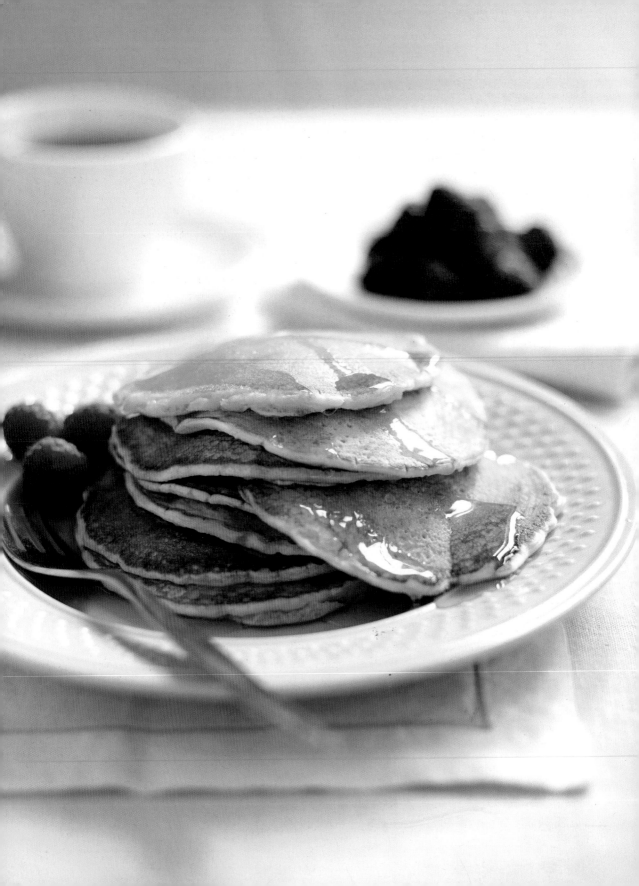

American pancakes

My image of the great American breakfast is hot, fresh coffee plus a stack of pancakes with soft brown crusts and a light inner sponge that soaks up honey, or maple or golden syrup so well. You can add more toppings – fresh fruits or soft dried fruit and a squeeze of lemon to cut through the sweetness – or even cream cheese or crumbled cooked bacon.

 ## nut free

125g (4½oz) plain flour
pinch of salt
2 tsp baking powder
2 tbsp caster sugar
1 large egg, beaten
200ml (7fl oz) milk
nut-free vegetable oil for frying
to serve
maple or golden syrup
handful of raspberries (optional)
lemon wedges (optional)

PREPARATION TIME 5 minutes
COOKING TIME 20 minutes
MAKES 8

1 Sift the flour with the salt, baking powder, and sugar.
2 Make a well in the centre, add the egg and half the milk and whisk (but do not overmix) to form a smooth, creamy batter. Stir in the remaining milk.
3 Heat a little oil in a frying pan over a medium heat. Pour off the excess. Add enough batter to the pan to make a pancake about 12cm (5in) in diameter, and cook until bubbles appear and pop on the surface and the pancake is almost set and brown underneath, about 1½ minutes. Flip it over with a palette knife and quickly cook the other side. Slide it out onto a plate and keep warm while you cook the remainder. Heat the pan with a little more oil between each pancake. If you have a big pan, you could cook 2–3 pancakes at a time.
4 Serve the pancakes hot with maple or golden syrup, raspberries, or lemon wedges to squeeze over.

TIP The pancakes are best made fresh so keep them warm on a plate over a pan of gently simmering water while you cook the remainder.

 ## dairy free
also nut free

Follow the recipe on the left, but use soya, rice, or oat milk in place of the cow's milk.

 ## egg free
also nut free

Follow the recipe on the left, but in step 1, whisk 1 tablespoon of potato flour with ¼ teaspoon of xanthan gum and 2 tablespoons of water until thick and frothy and add to the flour. In step 2, omit the egg and add an extra 3–4 tablespoons of milk to form a creamy consistency. Continue with steps 3 and 4, left.
◁ Pictured opposite

 ## gluten free
also nut free

Follow the recipe on the left, but use 55g (2oz) buckwheat flour and 55g (2oz) gluten-free plain white flour instead of plain flour.

Corned beef hash

Golden-brown, crispy fried potatoes are a great easy-to-cook breakfast or brunch meal. Partner them with salt beef for the famous deli speciality Corned beef hash or, more simply, cook Hash browns (see variation). Whichever you choose, it feeds a crowd and doesn't need split-second timing. There are endless additions and variations, my favourite is Red flannel hash served with lots of chopped parsley.

    dairy, egg, gluten & nut free

4 tbsp flavourless nut-free oil
1 large onion, finely chopped
450g (1lb) red-skinned or
   all-purpose potatoes, cooked,
   and cut into 1cm (½in) cubes
340g (12oz) corned beef, cut into
   1cm (½in) cubes
salt and freshly ground black
   pepper
1 tbsp Worcestershire sauce
   (optional)
chopped fresh parsley

PREPARATION TIME 25 minutes
COOKING TIME 10–15 minutes
SERVES 6

WATCH OUT FOR Worcestershire sauce as it can contain gluten. Make sure you use a gluten-free version.

VARIATIONS Add 2–3 chopped, cooked beetroots to the recipe at step 2 for a tasty Red flannel hash.
   For Hash browns, prepare as for the recipe on the left, but use 800g (1¾lb) of potatoes and omit the corned beef and Worcestershire sauce. At step 3, when the hash browns are golden brown underneath, use a spatula to flip them as a single "cake", or cut it into halves or quarters and turn. If needed, sprinkle a few more drops of oil into the pan. When golden brown on both sides, the hash browns are ready to serve. Popular additions to hash browns include diced green peppers, bacon, cheese (but not for dairy-sensitives), and fresh chopped chillies, but note the caution (left).

1 Heat the oil in a heavy-based frying pan and fry the onions over a fairly high heat, stirring occasionally, until lightly browned and turning crispy at the edges (about 4 minutes).
2 Add the cubed potatoes and corned beef and toss a few times to coat evenly in oil. Season with salt and pepper and sprinkle with Worcestershire sauce, if using.
3 Reduce the heat to moderate. Spread the potatoes and corned beef out in the pan and press down with a large spatula or fish slice. Cook for 10–15 minutes on a gentle heat until the bottom is brown and crispy – be careful not to cook it too quickly or it will burn.
4 Sprinkle the hash with the chopped fresh parsley, cut into wedges, and serve hot.

SERVING SUGGESTIONS Serve with poached or fried eggs (if eggs are tolerated). It is also delicious with chilli sauce or tomato ketchup, but be aware that some people cannot tolerate chilli and some bottled tomato ketchups are not suitable for people sensitive to gluten.

Smoothies

One of the most popular new breakfast foods, a good smoothie needs a balance of fruit, creaminess, and sweetness. As more people are enjoying dairy-free milks for taste and health reasons, even if they can eat dairy, I've used soya and oat milks as well as cow's milk and yogurt. Follow my recipes or create your own combinations with whatever ingredients you have to hand.

 egg free

banana oatie
1 large banana, chopped
240ml (8fl oz) oat milk
240ml (8fl oz) orange juice
55g (2oz) ground almonds
1 tbsp clear honey
ground cinnamon to dust

apricot & mango
170g (6oz) canned apricot
 halves, chopped
4 tbsp syrup from canned
 apricots
½ mango, chopped
240ml (8fl oz) orange juice
240ml (8fl oz) soya yogurt
½ tsp vanilla extract
squeeze of lime juice
handful of ice cubes

melon, grape & pear
170g (6oz) Galia melon (or other
 melon), chopped
2 pears, peeled and chopped
240ml (8fl oz) grape juice
2 ice cubes
mint sprig to garnish

mixed berry
170g (6oz) mixed red soft fruit
240ml (8fl oz) Greek yogurt
120ml (4fl oz) milk
2 ice cubes
3 tbsp clear honey

raspberry coulis (optional)
55g (2oz) raspberries
2 tbsp icing sugar

PREPARATION TIME 3–5 minutes
SERVES 1–2 (each smoothie)

 dairy free
also egg free

The smoothies are dairy free except for the mixed berry. Prepare as for the recipe on the left, but replace the yogurt and milk with soya or other dairy-free alternatives.

 gluten free
also egg free

The smoothies are gluten free except for the banana oatie. Prepare as for the recipe on the left, but replace the oat milk with any gluten-free milk.

 nut free
also egg free

The smoothies are nut free except for the banana oatie. Prepare as for the recipe on the left, but replace the almonds with 60ml (2fl oz) of coconut milk and reduce the oat milk to 120ml (4fl oz).

1 Put all the ingredients in a blender and blend until smooth. For a thick shake, add ice cubes before blending.
2 Pour into glasses and garnish. Serve as soon as possible.
3 For the raspberry coulis, mix the raspberries with the icing sugar, and press through a sieve. Swirl the coulis on top of each glass just before serving.
Pictured on next page ▶

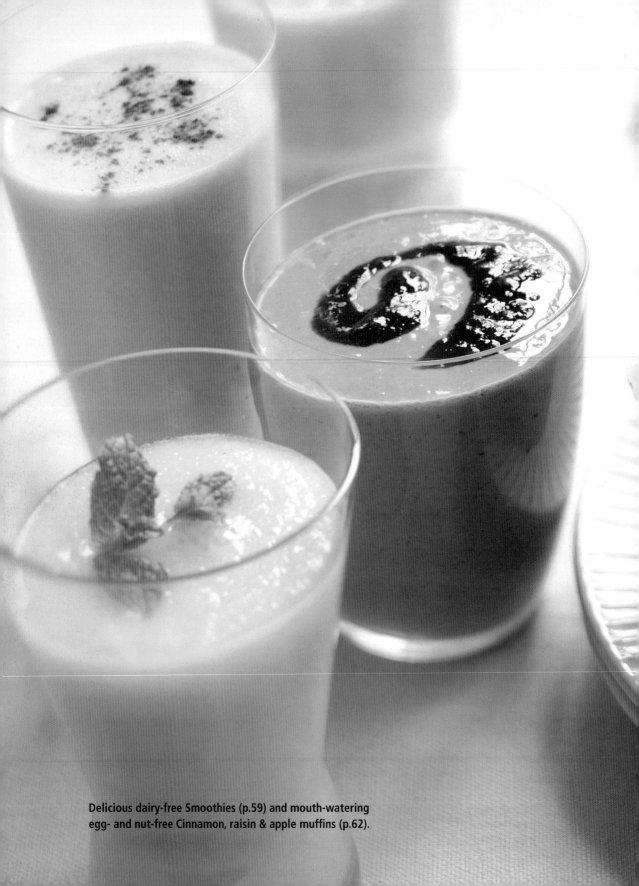

Delicious dairy-free Smoothies (p.59) and mouth-watering egg- and nut-free Cinnamon, raisin & apple muffins (p.62).

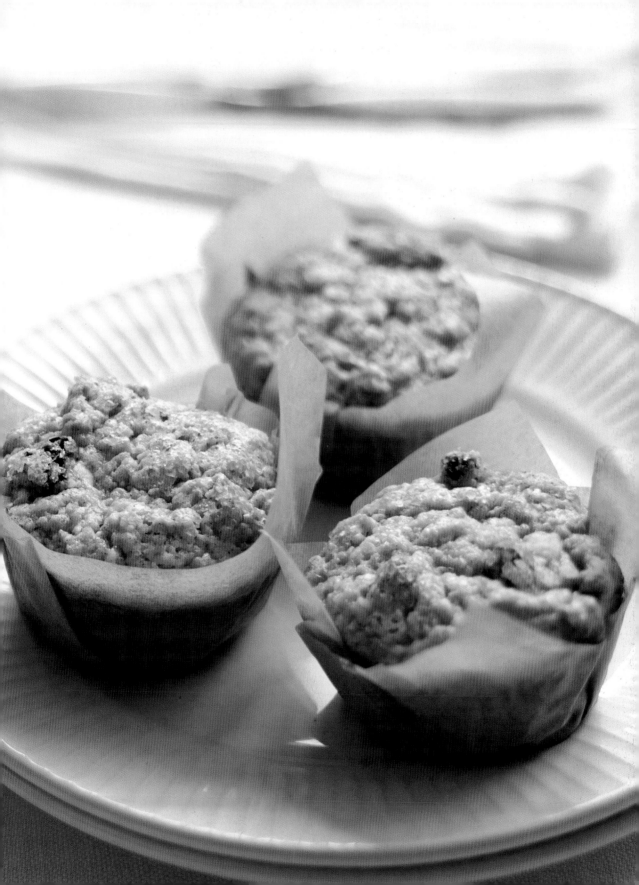

Cinnamon, raisin & apple muffins

There's a delicious cinnamon aroma from these as they bake and, from time to time, you'll catch a whiff of apple, too. Popular with all ages, the muffins have a lovely texture and are particularly good eaten warm for breakfast, but are also ideal as part of a packed lunch. You can even treat them as a tea bread and serve them split and buttered.

  ## egg & nut free

225g (8oz) plain flour
pinch of salt
1 tbsp baking powder
1 tsp ground cinnamon
45g (1½oz) soft brown sugar
45g (1½oz) butter or margarine,
  melted
2 apples, unpeeled and grated
55g (2oz) raisins
175ml (6fl oz) milk
demerara sugar to sprinkle
  (optional)

PREPARATION TIME 8 minutes
COOKING TIME 20 minutes
MAKES 12 muffins

1 Line 12 sections of a cake tin with medium-sized paper cases or grease the tins well. Preheat the oven to 200°C (400°F, gas 6).
2 Sift the flour, salt, baking powder, and cinnamon into a bowl.
3 Add the remaining ingredients and mix well. You will have a thick, wet dough.
4 Spoon into the prepared tins or cases (they should be full). Bake in the oven until risen, pale golden, and firm to the touch, about 20 minutes.
5 Transfer to a wire rack to cool.
◀ **Pictured on previous page**

TIP These muffins keep well for a few days in an airtight container and can also be frozen.

 ## dairy free
also egg & nut free

Follow the recipe on the left, but substitute dairy-free spread for the butter or ordinary margarine, and soya, rice, or oat milk for the cow's milk.

 ## gluten free
also egg & nut free

Follow the recipe on the left, but substitute gluten-free plain white flour for the ordinary flour and make sure the baking powder is gluten-free too. Add an extra 4 tablespoons of milk in step 3.

"A wonderful breakfast treat if you usually have to turn them down"

Blueberry muffins

For many, the blueberry muffin reigns supreme. Quick and easy to make, these light vanilla-flavoured cakes are oozing with juicy fruit. They are an excellent weekend treat for breakfast or a mid-morning snack and are ideally eaten fresh from the oven. We've been known to take an egg- and nut-free batch to our local coffee shop, so the whole family can enjoy coffee and muffins together.

 nut free

55g (2oz) butter or margarine
225g (8oz) plain flour
1 tbsp baking powder
pinch of salt
55g (2oz) caster sugar plus extra
   for dusting (optional)
150ml (5fl oz) milk
2 tsp lemon juice
½ tsp vanilla extract
1 egg, beaten
100g (3½oz) blueberries
ground cinnamon for dusting
   (optional)

PREPARATION TIME 15 minutes
COOKING TIME 20 minutes
MAKES 6 large or 10 small muffins

1 Line 6 large or 10 small muffin tin sections with paper cases or grease the tins well. Preheat the oven to 200°C (400°F, gas 6).
2 Melt the butter or margarine in a saucepan. Remove from the heat and leave to cool.
3 Sift the flour, baking powder, and salt into a bowl. Stir in the sugar.
4 Make a well in the centre, pour in the milk, lemon juice, vanilla extract, and egg. Fold the mixture quickly to combine, but don't worry if there are a few lumps. Fold the blueberries carefully into the mixture.
5 Spoon the mixture into the prepared tins (they will be almost full).
6 If liked, sprinkle lightly with cinnamon and sugar.
7 Bake in the oven until risen, lightly golden in colour, and the centres spring back when lightly pressed, about 25 minutes. Transfer to a wire rack, dust with caster sugar, and leave to cool.

 dairy free
also nut free

Follow the recipe on the left, but substitute dairy-free spread for the butter or ordinary margarine and soya, rice, or oat milk for the cow's milk.

 egg free
also nut free

Follow the recipe on the left, but substitute 1 tablespoon of potato flour mixed with 3 tablespoons of water for the beaten egg. The egg-free muffins will be slightly paler and smoother on top, but equally delicious.

 gluten free
also nut free

Follow the recipe on the left, but substitute gluten-free plain white flour for the ordinary plain flour and check that the baking powder is gluten free. Add an extra 4 tablespoons of milk.

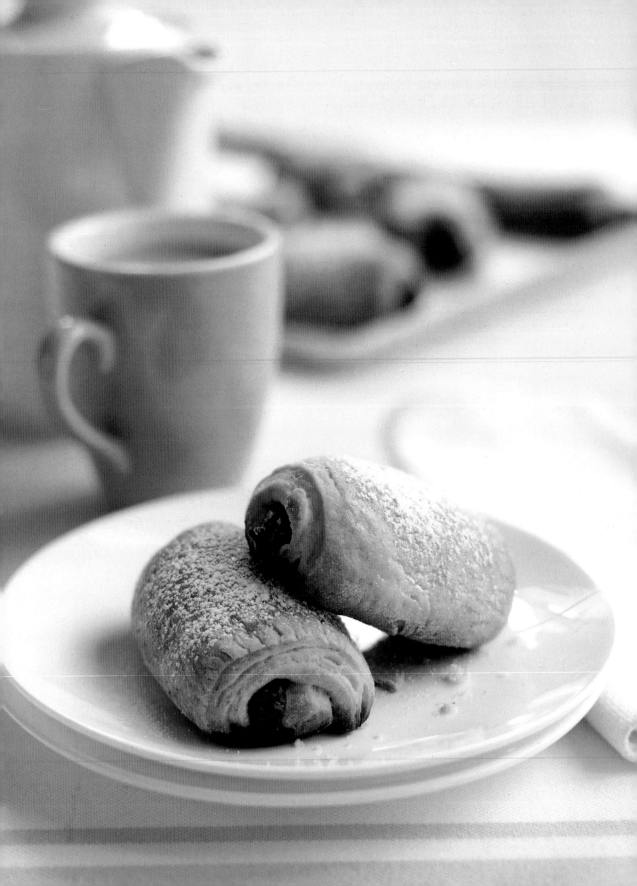

Pain au chocolat

Although these are a little fiddly to make, they are so delicious for breakfast with a cup of freshly brewed coffee and a glass of orange juice, you'll be glad you did. As they are especially popular with children, you could make a batch or two in advance to freeze until you need them. Nicest eaten freshly baked, pains au chocolat can be warmed briefly in a microwave or oven to serve.

 ## nut free

225g (8oz) strong plain flour,
   plus extra for dusting
1 tsp salt
2 tsp caster sugar
2 tsp fast-action dried yeast
85g (3oz) cold butter
105ml (7 tbsp) milk
1 egg, beaten
nut-free vegetable oil for greasing
to finish
1 egg
1 tsp icing sugar plus extra for
   dusting

24 squares of nut-free plain
   chocolate

PREPARATION TIME 30 minutes
   plus chilling and proving time
COOKING TIME 15 minutes
MAKES 8

1 Follow steps 1–5 of the nut-free croissant recipe on page 55.
2 Unwrap the dough, roll out on a floured surface again to a rectangle, but without adding butter. Fold as before, turn, roll, and fold again.
3 Dusting your rolling pin with flour, roll out the dough into a large rectangle, twice as long as it is high and about 5mm (¼ in) thick. Trim the edges and cut into 8 equal squares.
4 Grease a large baking sheet.
5 Beat the egg with the icing sugar and brush all over the surfaces of the squares. Put 3 squares of chocolate side by side on each square of dough. Fold the dough over the filling, so you can just see the chocolate at each end, and place on the baking sheets, sealed sides down.
6 Cover loosely with oiled cling film and leave in a warm place to prove until doubled in bulk, about 40 minutes.
7 Meanwhile, preheat the oven to 220°C (425°F, gas 7). Bake until puffy and golden, about 15 minutes.
8 Transfer to a wire rack to cool. Dust with a little sifted icing sugar. Best served warm.
◀ **Pictured opposite**

 ## dairy free
also nut free

Follow the nut-free recipe, but substitute hard white vegetable fat for the butter and use dairy-free chocolate.

 ## egg free
also nut free

Follow the nut-free recipe, but omit the egg. Add an extra 2–3 tablespoons of milk, if necessary. Use 3 tablespoons of single cream (or soya alternative to single cream) and 1 teaspoon of icing sugar for the glaze instead of the egg and icing sugar.

 ## gluten free

See overleaf for gluten-free recipe.

Pain au chocolat continued

 gluten free

225g (8oz) gluten-free plain white
   flour plus extra for dusting
½ tsp salt
2 tsp caster sugar
2 tsp xanthan gum
1 tbsp fast-action dried yeast
55g (2oz) cold butter, cut into
   1cm (½in) dice
150ml (5fl oz) milk
1 egg
a little vegetable oil for greasing

to finish
1 egg, beaten
1 tsp icing sugar plus extra for dusting
18 squares plain chocolate

PREPARATION TIME 25 minutes
COOKING TIME 15 minutes
MAKES 6

1 Follow steps 1–4 of the gluten-free croissant recipe on page 54.
2 Cut into 6 equal squares.
3 Grease a baking sheet.
4 Beat the egg with the icing sugar and brush all over the surfaces
  of the squares. Lay 3 squares of chocolate in the centre of the
  dough in a line. Fold over the dough and place, fold sides down,
  on the baking sheet. Cover loosely with oiled cling film and
  leave in a warm place to prove until well risen, about 45 minutes.
5 Meanwhile, preheat the oven to 200°C (400°F, gas 6). Brush the
  pains au chocolat with the remaining glaze. Bake until spongy
  and golden, about 15 minutes.
6 Dust with a little icing sugar. Best served warm or transfer to
  a wire rack to cool before wrapping and storing.

TIP These don't look as puffy as the wheat-based version, but they
are spongy, buttery, chocolatey, and delicious. Eat them warm, either
freshly baked or heated very briefly in the microwave or the oven.

Kedgeree

People get nostalgic about the country house appeal of this traditional breakfast dish of rice, fish, and eggs in a lightly curried sauce – but it also makes a great lunch or supper dish, especially with green vegetables or salad to accompany it. The lentils were in the original Indian dish adapted by the British and I've reinstated them as a healthy and tasty option.

  gluten & nut free

30g (1oz) green or brown lentils
   (optional)
250g (9oz) undyed smoked
   haddock or other smoked fish
300ml (10fl oz) milk
2 tbsp flavourless nut-free oil
1 onion, chopped
225g (8oz) long-grain rice
¾ tsp curry powder
¼ tsp ground turmeric
2 eggs

4 tbsp double cream
2 tsp lemon juice
salt and freshly ground black pepper
3 tbsp chopped fresh parsley

PREPARATION TIME 10 minutes
COOKING TIME 17 minutes plus
   lentils cooking time, if using
SERVES 4

1 If using, cook the lentils according to the packet instructions. When cooked, drain and set aside.
2 Poach the fish in the milk in a saucepan until it flakes easily with a fork, about 5 minutes. Lift the fish out and flake, discarding any skin and bones. Reserve the milk for the rice if you like your kedgeree with plenty of fishy flavour.
3 Heat the oil in a frying pan and fry the onion until softened but not browned, 2 minutes. Stir in the rice and spices until coated in the oil.
4 Measure 450ml (15fl oz) of liquid in a measuring jug. Use the poaching milk, topped up with boiling water, or just use boiling water. Pour onto the rice, onion, and spice mixture. Bring to the boil, stirring. Reduce the heat to low, stir once, and cover the pan. Cook the rice for 10 minutes or until all the liquid is absorbed and the rice is cooked, but not mushy. Fluff the rice with a fork and keep warm.
6 Meanwhile, in a separate saucepan, boil some water, reduce to a simmer, add the eggs, and cook for 5–7 minutes. Plunge the eggs immediately into cold water until cooled. Peel and cut into quarters.
7 Mix the fish and lentils, if using, into the rice with a fork. Stir in the cream and lemon juice. Gently fold in the egg, season to taste, and heat through very gently.
8 Garnish with chopped parsley before serving.

 dairy free
also gluten & nut free

Follow the recipe on the left, but substitute soya, rice, or oat milk (as long as there are no sensitivities to gluten) for the cow's milk and soya cream for the double cream.

 egg free
also gluten & nut free

Follow the recipe on the left, omitting the eggs and substituting 85g (3oz) of firm tofu – cut into 2.5cm (1in) pieces and steamed for 5 minutes. Alternatively, use 4 large scallops, sliced horizontally into two or three pieces, and brushed with a thin film of oil. Sauté the scallop slices in a hot pan until just cooked but still soft, 30 seconds to 1 minute, and add in step 7 instead of the eggs.

TIP Garnish with coriander leaves instead of parsley, if liked.

Tortillas

Tortillas are so versatile; use them to scoop up Chilli con carne (p.122), wrap around fillings for lunchbox treats, or turn stale ones into tortilla chips to serve with dips (p.70). Mexican cooks make small tortillas by pressing out balls of *masa harina* (ground corn) and water – but this can be quite fiddly to do. This batter-based version makes lovely, soft, rollable tortillas.

  dairy & nut free

55g (2oz) plain flour
55g (2oz) maize meal
pinch of salt
1 large egg, beaten
150ml (5fl oz) water

PREPARATION TIME 5 minutes
COOKING TIME 20 minutes
MAKES 8

1 Mix the dry ingredients together in a bowl.
2 Beat in the egg and water to form a fairly thin batter. Pour into a measuring jug.
3 Dust a sheet of kitchen paper with flour on the work surface.
4 Heat a small, non-stick heavy frying pan. Reduce the heat to moderate.
5 Pour in an eighth of the batter and lift the pan up to quickly swirl the batter round the pan to coat the base and a little way up the sides. Cook over a moderate heat until the edge of the tortilla begins to curl slightly. Flip over and quickly dry out the other side.
6 Slide onto the kitchen paper and dust with a little more flour. Cover with a second sheet of kitchen paper to keep the tortilla soft. Repeat, reheating the pan slightly between each tortilla, and stirring the batter every time. If you're not planning to use the tortillas straight away, cool them, and store in an airtight container. They are suitable for freezing.
7 See the serving suggestion on the right for delicious lunchtime wrap ideas.
   Pictured opposite ▶

 egg free
also dairy & nut free

Follow the recipe on the left, but omit the egg and substitute 30g (1oz) of potato flour for half of the maize meal and increase the water to 240ml (8fl oz).

 gluten free
also dairy & nut free

Follow the recipe on the left, but substitute gluten-free plain flour for the ordinary plain flour and increase the water to 215ml (7½ fl oz).

SERVING SUGGESTION Try the following ideas for lunchbox wraps. For herb dip with roasted peppers, use the Herb dip recipe on page 71. Spread generously onto a tortilla, add a handful of roasted peppers, and roll up into a wrap.

For smoked salmon with crème fraîche, spread some crème fraîche (or, if you can't tolerate dairy, soya cream cheese thinned with soya cream and a squeeze of lemon) onto a tortilla. Add a slice of smoked salmon and roll up into a wrap.

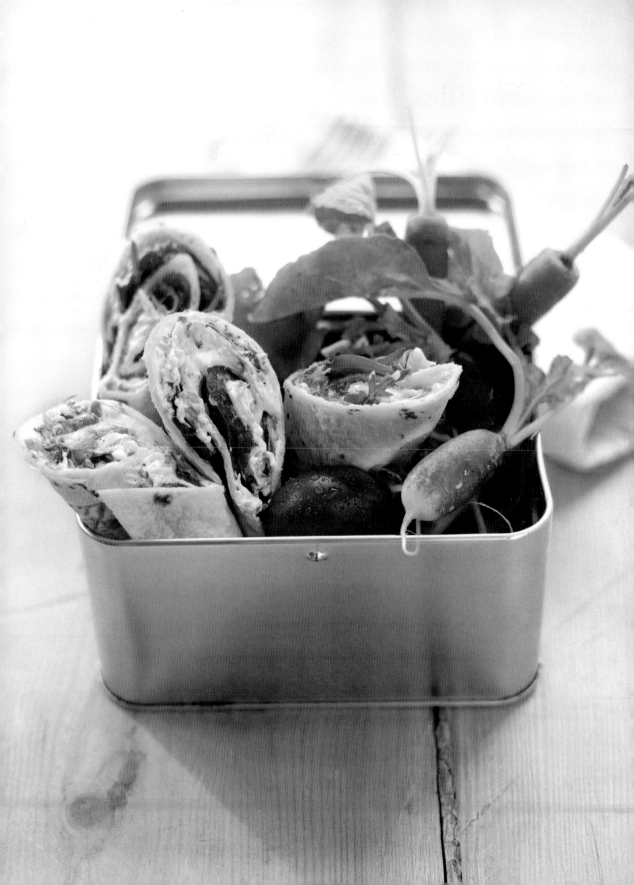

Tortilla chips

It's worthwhile making your own tortilla chips because, although shop-bought tortilla chips may be gluten and egg free, some may contain traces of nuts or milk powder, so aren't suitable for everyone. They are also really easy to make using the tortilla recipe that suits you on page 68. In Mexico, tortillas are made every day and any leftover stale ones are fried to serve with dips – so they're never wasted.

    dairy, egg, gluten & nut free

1 quantity stale tortillas in
   appropriate version (p.68)
nut-free vegetable oil for frying
salt (optional)
for the salsa
1 ripe avocado, pitted and finely
   diced
juice of 1 lime
1 small onion, finely chopped
1 green pepper, finely diced
1 red chilli, deseeded and finely
   chopped

2 tbsp olive oil
pinch of caster sugar
2 tbsp chopped fresh coriander
freshly ground black pepper

PREPARATION TIME 2 minutes
COOKING TIME 8 minutes
SERVES 4

1 Cut each tortilla into 6 wedges.
2 Heat about 5mm (¼in) of oil in a frying pan.
3 Add the tortilla wedges a few at a time and fry, turning once or twice until crisp and golden, 1–2 minutes. Remove with a draining spoon and drain on kitchen paper.
4 Repeat until all the chips are cooked. Sprinkle with salt, if liked, and leave to cool.
5 Mix all the salsa ingredients together and transfer to a small pot. Place on a large plate and surround with the tortilla chips.

WATCH OUT FOR chillies, as some people are sensitive to them.

SERVING SUGGESTION For nachos, top tortilla chips with grated cheese (or a dairy-free melting variety) and chopped mild green Jalapeño peppers (if tolerated) and grill until the cheese has melted.

"Serve these at a party – and you can be sure that absolutely all your guests can dip in"

Herb dip

This garlic herb dip has a fresh summery taste that is perfect for serving with crisp crudités and is equally delicious as a snack on toasted brown bread. An excellent idea for a buffet is to use the herb dip as a topping on halved cherry tomatoes or baked new potatoes, scattered with a little sea salt. Vary the green herbs according to what you have available.

   egg, gluten & nut free

200g (7oz) plain Greek-style
  yogurt or soured cream
225g (8oz) cream cheese
2 tbsp olive oil
grated zest and juice of ½ lemon
1 small garlic clove, skinned
  and crushed
2 tbsp finely chopped fresh
  parsley
1 tbsp finely chopped fresh basil
1 tbsp finely chopped fresh
  chervil
4 spring onions, finely chopped
salt and freshly ground black
  pepper to taste

PREPARATION TIME 5 minutes
SERVES 4

1 Place all the ingredients in a food processor or blender and pulse until well blended. Season the dip to taste.
2 Serve chilled with crudités, tortilla chips, or crisps. This dip also makes a delicious filling for tortilla wraps (p.68).
3 This dip can be stored, covered, in a refrigerator for up to a day.

TIP This recipe makes enough to top 20 baked new potatoes or cherry tomato halves.

 dairy free
also egg, gluten & nut free

Follow the recipe on the left, but substitute soya-based yogurt for the yogurt or soured cream and replace the cream cheese with soya-based cream cheese alternative or silken tofu. Reduce the olive oil to 1 tablespoon, as the dairy-free version needs less liquid.

SIDE DISHES, STARTERS & LIGHT MEALS

Crostini & toppings

Literally "little toasts", crostini are slices of bread, rubbed with garlic, brushed with olive oil, and then toasted. Served as starters or snacks, they work best with gutsy Mediterranean flavours as toppings, such as olives, aubergines, tomatoes, basil, and peppers. If you can't buy Italian or French bread to suit you, use the recipes for French-style bread (pp.170–71) or Focaccia (p.173).

    dairy, egg, gluten & nut free

aubergine & mushroom

4 tbsp olive oil plus extra for brushing
1 shallot, finely chopped
1 aubergine, finely diced
½ tsp ground cumin
½ tsp ground cinnamon
½ tsp dried oregano
55g (2oz) button mushrooms, thinly sliced
salt and freshly ground black pepper
1 tbsp chopped fresh parsley

8 diagonal slices of allergen-free French-style bread (pp.170–71) or half slices of Focaccia (p.173)
2 garlic cloves, halved

PREPARATION TIME 10 minutes
COOKING TIME 6 minutes
MAKES 8

SERVING SUGGESTION Try crumbling a little feta cheese or dairy-free alternative over the aubergine mixture before serving.

1 Heat the oil in a saucepan. Add the shallot and aubergine and fry over a fairly gentle heat until almost soft, about 4 minutes. Add the spices, oregano, and mushrooms and fry for a further 2 minutes, stirring all the time. Season and stir in the parsley.
2 Meanwhile, rub the bread all over with garlic, brush both sides with olive oil and then toast.
3 Pile the aubergine and mushroom mixture on the toast and serve.

tomato & sweet basil

4 tomatoes, deseeded and chopped
1 tbsp olive oil plus extra for brushing
few chopped fresh basil leaves
freshly ground black pepper
8 diagonal slices of allergen-free

French-style bread (pp.170–71) or half slices of Focaccia (p.173)
1 large garlic clove, halved

PREPARATION TIME 5 minutes
COOKING TIME 3–4 minutes
MAKES 8

1 Mix the tomatoes with the oil, basil leaves, and a good grinding of black pepper.
2 Meanwhile, toast the bread as above.
3 Place on a serving platter and spoon the tomato mixture on top.

tapenade

120ml (4fl oz) olive oil plus
    extra for brushing
115g (4oz) pitted black olives
115g (4oz) pitted green olives
1 large garlic clove
3 tbsp chopped fresh parsley
2 tbsp capers in brine, rinsed
    and drained
1 x 55g (2oz) can of anchovy
    fillets, drained
juice of $\frac{1}{2}$ lime
$\frac{1}{4}$ tsp caster sugar
freshly ground black pepper

8 diagonal slices of allergen-free
    French-style bread (pp.170–71)
    or half slices of Focaccia (p.173)

to finish
1 small onion, very finely chopped
juice of $\frac{1}{2}$ lime

PREPARATION TIME 10 minutes
COOKING TIME 3–4 minutes
MAKES 8

TIP You can bake the bread in the oven, if you prefer. Lay the prepared slices of bread on a baking sheet and bake at 180°C (350°F, gas 4) for 15 minutes or until crisp and golden, turning once.

1 Put all the tapenade ingredients in a blender or food processor, adding a good grinding of pepper. Run the machine to form a coarse paste, stopping and scraping down the sides as necessary.

2 Mix the onion and lime juice and leave to stand for at least 1 hour.

3 Brush the bread with oil and then toast.

4 Top each slice with a spoonful of tapenade and sprinkle with the onion and lime juice.

pepper, courgette & sun-dried tomato

1 tbsp olive oil plus extra for
    brushing
2 shallots, finely chopped
1 small red or orange pepper,
    deseeded and chopped
1 courgette, chopped
1 tsp chopped fresh rosemary
2 tsp balsamic vinegar
salt and freshly ground black
    pepper

8 diagonal slices of allergen-free
    French-style bread (pp.170–71)
    or half slices of Focaccia (p.173)
1 garlic clove, halved
1 tbsp sun-dried tomato paste

PREPARATION TIME 15 minutes
COOKING TIME 7–8 minutes
MAKES 8

1 Heat the oil in a frying pan. Add the shallot, pepper, courgette, and rosemary and fry over a moderate heat, stirring, until just soft, about 4 minutes. Stir in the balsamic vinegar and a little salt and pepper.

2 Rub the bread all over with garlic, brush both sides with olive oil, and then toast.

3 Spread each slice with a little sun-dried tomato paste and spoon the warm pepper mixture on top. Serve warm.

SIDE DISHES, STARTERS & LIGHT MEALS

73

California temaki sushi

Here's sushi that is fun to make at home as it doesn't need to look perfect. Hand-rolled cones of nori (Japanese seaweed) are folded around fillings – like wrapping a bunch of flowers – and eaten with bowls of wasabi, soy sauce, and pickled ginger. Serve as an appetizer or increase the quantities and arrange the ingredients on dishes, for guests to assemble their own DIY party starter.

    dairy, egg, gluten & nut free

1 tbsp sushi vinegar
pinch of salt
1 tsp caster sugar
150g (5½oz) short-grain sushi
  rice, pre-washed
300ml (10fl oz) water
4 nori sheets, cut in half
¼ tsp wasabi paste
8 tsp appropriate version of
  Mayonnaise (p.210)
4 lettuce leaves, torn into 2.5cm
  (1in) pieces

8 large king prawns, cooked and peeled
8 tsp flying fish or salmon roe
5cm (2in) piece of cucumber,
  deseeded and cut into matchsticks
¼ avocado, cut into 8 slices and tossed
  in lemon juice to prevent browning

PREPARATION TIME 40 minutes
COOKING TIME 20 minutes
SERVES 8

VARIATIONS Alternative fillings include sushi quality raw fish, lightly steamed asparagus, thinly sliced carrots, shiitake or other mushrooms cooked in a soy-flavoured broth, crabsticks, spring onions, snow peas, fresh silken or deep fried tofu, and sesame seeds.

WATCH OUT FOR seafood allergies. Use non-seafood variations such as vegetables or tofu (as listed above). If serving with soy sauce, make sure it is gluten free if need be.

TIP See resources (pp. 218–219) for stockists of Japanese ingredients.

1 Mix the vinegar with the salt and sugar, stirring until dissolved.
2 Put the rice and water in a saucepan. Bring to the boil, stir, reduce the heat to as low as possible and cover and simmer very gently for 15–20 minutes or until the water has been absorbed and the rice is sticky. Remove from the heat and leave to stand, covered, for 10 minutes. Add the sushi vinegar mixture and fluff with a fork.
3 To assemble the maki, take a half sheet of nori and lay it rough side up across your left hand. Add 1 heaped tablespoon of rice to the left half of the nori sheet, covering half the sheet.
4 Mix the wasabi and mayonnaise. Take a teaspoon of wasabi mayonnaise and starting at the bottom left-hand corner, spread the mayonnaise in a diagonal line up to the top of the rice.
5 Place one piece of lettuce, one prawn, 1 teaspoon of roe, and a slice each of the cucumber and avocado, on the top of half the rice, to the mayonnaise line.
6 Gently but firmly, lift the bottom left corner of rice-covered nori and fold it up over the filling to the top right corner of rice, using your left thumb to help roll it over. It is important to be firm and to get the corners to meet. Then wrap the top right-hand corner of uncovered nori over, down and around the back to form a cone. Dampen the last corner with water to stick it to the cone.
7 Repeat for the remaining nori sheets.

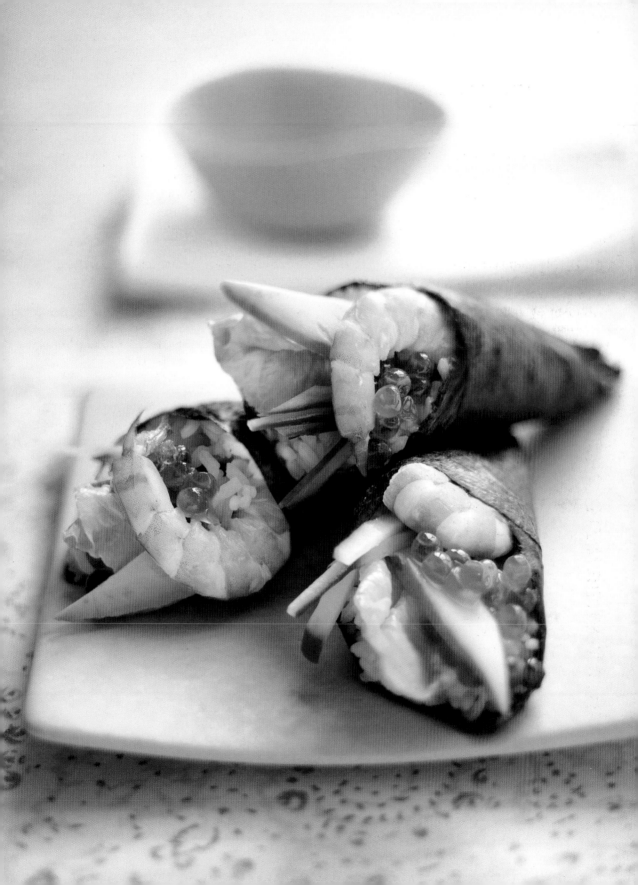

Blini with smoked salmon

These little buckwheat pancakes, an East European favourite, are traditionally served with soured cream, caviar, and chopped onion. Like the smoked salmon version below, they can be served as an elegant starter, garnished with dill sprigs. Buckwheat, which is a seed, despite its name, does not contain gluten and gives a darkish flour with a slightly nutty taste; mix half-and-half with regular flour if preferred.

   nut, egg & gluten free

for the pancakes
200g (7oz) buckwheat flour
1/4 tsp caster sugar
1/4 tsp salt
1 1/2 tsp fast-action dried yeast
30g (1oz) butter
450ml (15fl oz) milk
2 tbsp warm water
nut-free vegetable oil for frying
to finish
12 thin slices of smoked salmon
2–3 onions, finely chopped
150ml (5fl oz) soured cream

to garnish
fresh chive stalks
lemon wedges

PREPARATION TIME 10 minutes
   plus standing time
COOKING TIME 30 minutes
SERVES 6 (makes about 30)

1 Sift the flour, sugar, and salt into a fairly large bowl and stir in the yeast.
2 Melt the butter in a saucepan. Remove from the heat and add the milk. Stir. It should be comfortably warm to the touch.
3 Gradually beat the milk and butter mixture into the flour mixture to form a thick, creamy batter. Cover the bowl with oiled cling film and leave in a warm place until doubled in bulk, about 1 hour.
4 Beat again, then beat in the water to form a thick, creamy batter again.
5 Heat a little oil in a large heavy frying pan then pour off the excess. Put 3 separate tablespoonfuls of the batter well apart in the pan, swirling them gently with the tip of the spoon to make neat rounds, about 5cm (2in) in diameter. Fry until the pancakes dry out and bubbles appear and burst all over the surface. Flip them over and quickly cook the other sides. Slide onto a plate and keep warm over a pan of gently simmering water while you cook the remainder (the batter makes about 30).
6 Put several blini on each plate with 2 rolls of smoked salmon, a small pile of chopped onion, and a spoonful of soured cream. Garnish with a wedge of lemon and a few chive stalks, and serve while the blini are still warm.

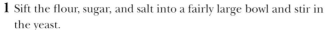 **dairy free**
also egg, gluten & nut free

Follow the recipe on the left, but substitute dairy-free spread for the butter and soya, rice, or oat milk for the cow's milk. Serve with dairy-free soured cream alternative, silken tofu, or plain soya yogurt instead of the soured cream.

TIP You may need to discard the first few blini as, like pancakes, these are the ones that prepare the pan for the successful ones to follow.

Three blini may be enough for a starter. The rest will freeze beautifully and then can be reheated on a plate over a pan of simmering water or in the microwave.

Chicken fajitas

A riot of mouth-watering Mexican flavours; chicken sizzled in cumin, chilli, and coriander, tossed with peppers, onions, and garlic and topped with cooling, creamy guacamole. Buy tortillas or make the right allergen-free tortilla for you (p.68), then roll the still sizzling filling into the warmed wraps. You can also, more traditionally, make these with strips of fried steak. Serve as an appetizer or a light meal.

    dairy, egg, gluten & nut free

for the fajitas
3 tbsp olive oil
1 red onion, halved and sliced
1 garlic clove, crushed
2 large red peppers, halved, deseeded and cut into strips
2 large green peppers, halved, deseeded and cut into strips
4 tomatoes, cut into wedges
4 skinless chicken breasts, cut into strips
1/4 tsp chilli powder
1/2 tsp ground cumin
1/2 tsp ground coriander
1/2 tsp dried oregano

for the guacamole
1 large ripe avocado, halved and pitted
juice of 1/2 lemon
2 tbsp snipped fresh chives
salt and freshly ground black pepper
few drops of Tabasco (optional)
to serve
8 tortillas (p.68)
large green salad

PREPARATION TIME 20 minutes
COOKING TIME 8 minutes
SERVES 4

1 To make the guacamole, scoop the flesh of the avocado into a small bowl and mash with the lemon and chives and season to taste. Add a few drops of Tabasco, if liked, for added fire.
2 Heat the oil in a frying pan or wok. Add the onion, garlic, peppers, and tomatoes and stir-fry until nearly tender, about 4 minutes. Add the chicken and stir-fry for 2 minutes. Stir in the spices and herbs and season to taste.
3 Meanwhile, warm the tortillas on a covered plate over a pan of simmering water or wrap them in kitchen paper and warm briefly in the microwave.
4 To serve, divide the chicken mixture amongst the tortillas, top each with a spoonful of guacamole and roll up. Place, rolled sides down, on warm plates and serve with a large green salad.

SERVING SUGGESTION Instead of guacamole, you may like to top the fajita filling with a spoonful of soured cream or plain yogurt. Use a dairy-free soured cream alternative or yogurt, if necessary. You can also add some shredded lettuce and grated Cheddar cheese (or dairy-free Cheddar alternative).

WATCH OUT FOR chillies as some people can't tolerate them. Omit the chilli powder if in any doubt.

SIDE DISHES, STARTERS & LIGHT MEALS

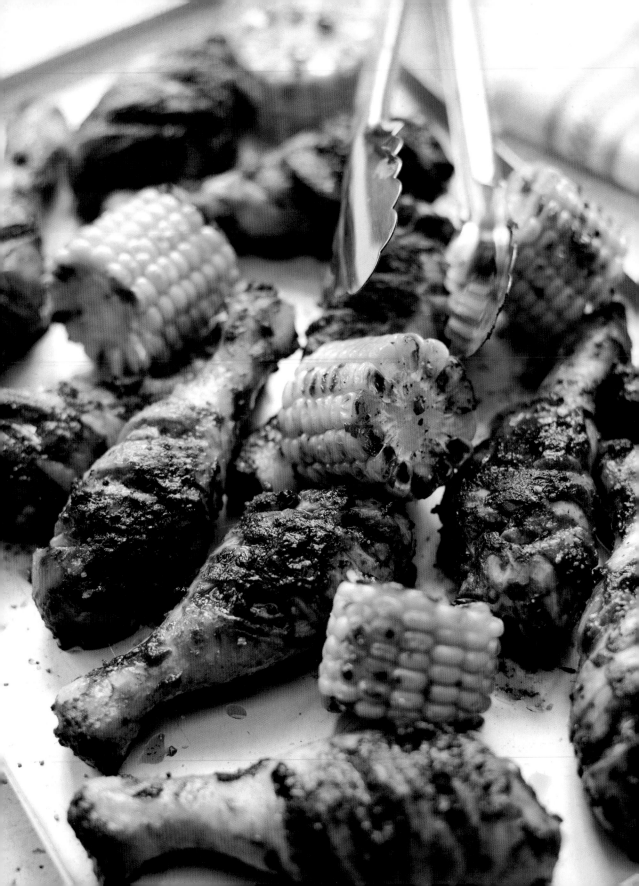

Chicken drumsticks

A really useful recipe, popular with all ages, these chicken drumsticks can feed a crowd and you'll have none of the "Big Four" allergens to worry about. They are great for lunch or dinner and ideal for barbecues, especially if serving with grilled corn. Add a baked potato for a filling and nutritious meal. The easy-to-make barbecue sauce scores over shop-bought versions as it contains neither wheat nor dairy.

   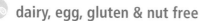 **dairy, egg, gluten & nut free**

3 tbsp corn or other flavourless
  nut-free oil
2 tbsp molasses
4 tbsp tomato purée
1 tsp mustard powder
2 tbsp wine vinegar
2 tsp Worcestershire sauce
1/4 tsp smoked paprika (pimentón)
salt and freshly ground black
  pepper
8 chicken drumsticks

PREPARATION TIME 5 minutes
  plus chilling time
COOKING TIME 14–16 minutes
SERVES 4

1 Mix all the ingredients, apart from the drumsticks, in a shallow sealable container, seasoning well with salt and pepper.
2 Make several slashes in the flesh on each chicken leg before adding them to the marinade – this lets the flavour in and also helps them to cook more evenly. Turn the chicken drumsticks to coat them thoroughly.
3 Cover and chill for at least 4 hours or overnight.
4 Remove the chicken from the marinade and shake off the excess.
5 Cook under a preheated grill or on the barbecue for 7–8 minutes on each side or until richly browned and the juices run clear when a skewer is inserted into the thickest part of the meat.

WATCH OUT FOR mustard powder, Worcestershire sauce, and paprika – check that they are gluten free, if need be.

SERVING SUGGESTION These are delicious served with grilled corn on the cob. Roll the cobs in a mixture of salt, pepper, and chillies, with lime squeezed over, and cook under a grill or barbecue. Note that some people are sensitive to chillies, so omit if in any doubt.

"This is tasty, unpretentious finger food for the whole family to enjoy"

SIDE DISHES, STARTERS & LIGHT MEALS

Soy-honey glazed sausages

I've used cocktail sausages as an appetizer or party snack for this recipe, but if you use full-sized sausages it makes an excellent main course for a meal served with mustardy mashed potatoes, wilted greens and Vegetable gravy (p.215). Alternatively, serve the sausages with lentils or beans and fries for a failsafe, popular supper for children.

   dairy, egg & nut free

500g (1lb 2oz) cocktail sausages
1 tbsp soy sauce
1 tbsp clear honey
1 tbsp sesame seeds

PREPARATION TIME 2 minutes
COOKING TIME 30 minutes
SERVES 4

 gluten free
also dairy, egg & nut free

Use pure pork or other gluten-free sausages and a gluten-free soy sauce. If serving with mustard, check it is gluten free too.

1 Preheat the oven to 180°C (350°F, gas 4). Arrange the sausages in a single layer in a roasting tin and cook until just beginning to brown, 10 minutes.
2 Mix together the soy sauce and honey. Remove the sausages from the oven, spoon over the soy mixture and toss to coat. Return to the oven until glazed and browned, about 20 minutes. Turn once or twice during cooking.
3 Sprinkle with the sesame seeds and toss to coat before serving.

WATCH OUT FOR sesame seeds, as some people are allergic to them.

"Children love these sausages – the soy-glaze adds a barbecue flavour"

Grilled polenta

Use these polenta toasts as canapé bases or as a snack or starter with toppings such as Parmesan, rocket, and lightly steamed green vegetables; prosciutto; Pesto (p.211), or any of the toppings described in the Crostini recipe (pp.72–3). You can also stop halfway through this recipe for a soft, stirred version of polenta, which makes a great side dish for stews and casseroles.

   egg, gluten & nut free

400ml (14fl oz) water
1 tbsp olive oil plus extra for brushing
½ tsp salt
100g (3½oz) quick-cook polenta
salt and pepper to season
1 heaped tbsp grated Parmesan

PREPARATION TIME 20 minutes
COOKING TIME 4–5 minutes
SERVES 4

1 Place the water, olive oil, and salt in a medium-sized saucepan. Bring to the boil.
2 Add the polenta to the boiling water in a thin stream and stir constantly. Reduce the heat to a low simmer and cook, stirring constantly throughout, for 15 minutes or until the polenta has thickened. Add the grated Parmesan and stir to mix. Season to taste with salt and pepper. Remove from the heat.
3 Spoon the polenta onto a large flat plate or baking tray and spread it out evenly, smoothing it with the back of a large spoon, to form a circular cake about 2cm (¾in) thick. Leave to cool. You can store it at this stage in the refrigerator for up to a day.
4 To grill, cut the polenta cake into strips or wedges. Brush with a thin layer of olive oil and then grill or griddle until browned on both sides. Serve with a choice of toppings.

 dairy free
also egg, gluten & nut free

Replace the Parmesan with an equal quantity of dairy-free cheese. I have tried it with both dairy-free Parmesan and dairy-free Cheddar and they both work well – though the Parmesan can be a little salty.

VARIATION For a soft, stirred version of polenta, just stop at the end of step 2. As well as working well with stews and dishes that have lots of sauce or juice, this is a classic accompaniment to Osso bucco (p.118).

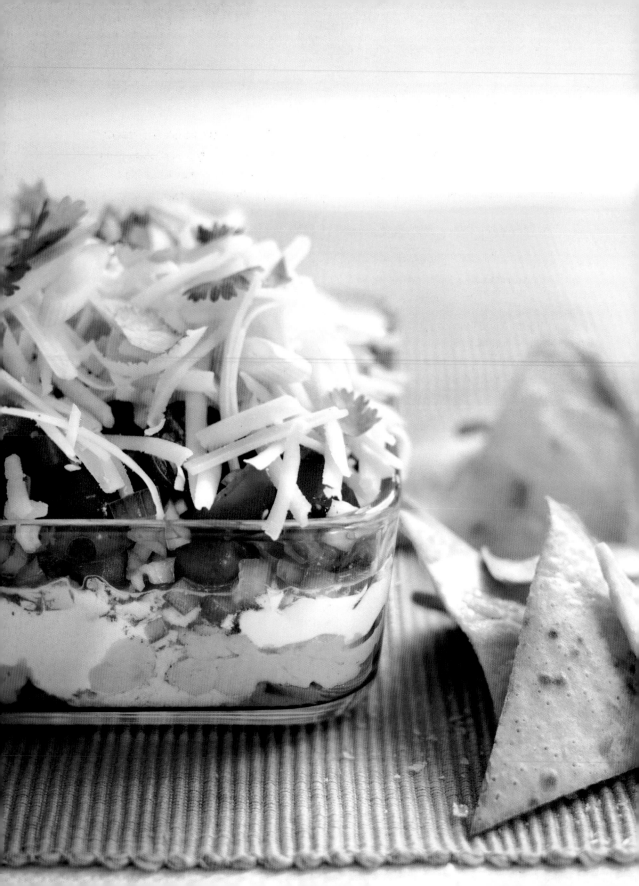

Seven-layer dip

This is an unabashed and lavish layered party dip that is a riot of colours and flavours. It looks stunning served in a deep glass dish. For a speedier version, follow the recipe, but use ready-made guacamole in place of the avocados and shop-bought salsa for the tomatoes, or take a little longer to make the mouth-watering fresh version below. Serve with Tortilla chips (p.70) or toasted flatbreads.

   egg, gluten & nut free

3 avocados
juice of 1 lime or lemon
450g (1lb) canned refried beans
500ml (17fl oz) soured cream
¼ tsp chilli powder
2 green peppers, deseeded and finely chopped
340g (12oz) drained pitted black olives, halved
8 tomatoes, chopped
½ red onion, chopped

750g (1lb 10oz) Cheddar or Monterey Jack cheese, coarsely grated
chopped fresh coriander and spring onions to garnish

PREPARATION TIME 20 minutes
SERVES 16–20

 dairy free
also egg, gluten & nut free

Follow the recipe on the left, but replace the soured cream with the same quantity of dairy-free soured cream or soya yogurt, and the Cheddar or Monterey Jack cheese with the same quantity of a non-dairy equivalent.

1 Peel and mash the avocados with the lime juice, using a fork.
2 To assemble, layer the refried beans over the base of a large glass dish. Add the mashed avocados and then the soured cream and sprinkle the chilli powder on top.
3 For the green pepper layer, sprinkle the chopped pepper around the perimeter of the dish first, to ensure that the layer is visible, and sprinkle the rest evenly over the centre. Layer the halved olives carefully on top and spoon over the chopped tomatoes and red onion. Finally, add the cheese and the coriander and spring onion garnish. Chill until ready to serve.

◀ **Pictured opposite**

WATCH OUT FOR chilli powder, as some people cannot tolerate it. Substitute with an equal quantity of ground cumin if this is a problem.

VARIATION If you like things spicier, add 3 tablespoons of chopped Jalapeño peppers to the green pepper layer and replace the chilli powder with 25g (1oz) of taco seasoning.

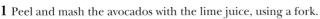

SIDE DISHES, STARTERS & LIGHT MEALS

Bacon & onion quiche

A baked dish of eggs and cream in a pastry crust is not an obvious recipe for this book! But here are four versions, each with crisp pastry shells and a creamy, slightly wobbly custard encasing the filling of bacon, onion, herbs, and cheese. Mix the filling well into the custard, and do add the mustard into the egg-free version – it makes all the difference.

 ## nut free

1 quantity of nut- and egg-free
   shortcrust pastry (p.180)
1 tbsp flavourless nut-free oil
2 onions, chopped
6 rashers streaky bacon,
   rinded and diced
3 eggs
360ml (12fl oz) single cream
115g (4oz) hard cheese, eg
   Cheddar, grated
2 tbsp chopped fresh parsley

1 tbsp chopped fresh sage
salt and freshly ground black pepper

PREPARATION TIME 30 minutes
   plus pastry chilling time
COOKING TIME 35 minutes
SERVES 6–8

1 Preheat the oven to 200°C (400°F, gas 6).
2 Roll out the pastry and use to line a 25cm (10in) flan dish.
  Place on a baking sheet. Prick the base with a fork and fill with
  crumpled foil or greaseproof paper and baking beans. Bake in
  the oven for 10 minutes. Remove the foil or paper and beans
  and bake for about 5 minutes, until lightly golden and dried
  out. Remove from the oven. Reduce the temperature to 190°C
  (375°F, gas 5).
3 Meanwhile, heat the oil in a frying pan and fry the onion for
  2 minutes, stirring, until translucent. Add the bacon and
  continue to fry for a further 2 minutes. Remove from the pan
  with a draining spoon and reserve.
4 Beat the eggs and cream together with half the cheese and
  herbs. Season with salt and pepper.
5 Transfer the bacon and onion mixture to the flan case and
  spread it evenly. Spoon over the egg and cream mixture.
  Sprinkle the remaining cheese on top. Bake in the oven for 35
  minutes until bubbling, set, and turning pale golden. Serve
  warm or cold.

 ## dairy free
also nut free

Follow the recipe on the left, but use the dairy-free Shortcrust pastry recipe (p.182). Use soya cream in place of the single cream and Cheddar-type soya cheese alternative instead of the Cheddar cheese.

 ## egg free
also nut free

Follow the recipe on the left, but omit the eggs. At step 4 put 6 tablespoons of potato flour in a bowl with 1½ teaspoons of xanthan gum and 200ml (7fl oz) water. Whisk with an electric beater until thick and white and the mixture stands in soft peaks. Whisk in the 360ml (12fl oz) of cream and a tablespoon of English or Dijon mustard. Beat together with half the cheese, the herbs, and salt and pepper to taste. Continue from step 5.

 ## gluten free
also nut free

Prepare as for the recipe on the left, but use the gluten-free Shortcrust pastry recipe on page 182.

Gazpacho

An easy-to-make chilled tomato soup, perfect for a hot summer day. Recipes vary depending on which region of Spain you find yourself in – this is based on the Andalucian version. Serve it in bowls with a garnish of finely chopped vegetables or in glasses, as they do in Spanish restaurants and bars. Gazpacho has been described as "liquid salad" and is every bit as healthy.

   ## dairy, egg & nut free

1kg (2¼lb) fresh ripe tomatoes, skinned and quartered
½ small onion, quartered
½ green or red pepper, deseeded and quartered
1 cucumber, peeled, deseeded and quartered
2 garlic cloves, peeled and halved
150ml (5fl oz) olive oil
1 small day-old bread roll or thick slice of bread (about 55g/2oz), soaked in water
3 tbsp wine vinegar
good pinch of sugar

½ red or green chilli, deseeded and chopped (optional)
salt and freshly ground black pepper
iced water to thin (optional)
to garnish
a selection of any of the following: small croûtons; finely diced tomatoes; red and green peppers; cucumber; onion; or chopped fresh parsley

PREPARATION TIME 15 minutes plus chilling time
SERVES 4–6

1 In a food processor blend together the tomatoes, onion, pepper, cucumber, garlic, olive oil, bread (squeeze out the water just before using), vinegar, sugar, and chilli, if using. Blend for 1 minute or until smooth. Season to taste with salt and pepper. Chill for at least 2 hours before serving and thin with iced water, if necessary.
2 Serve with your choice of garnish or arrange the garnish in small bowls at the table and allow guests to choose their own.

SERVING SUGGESTION If eggs are tolerated, a little very finely chopped hard boiled egg is an attractive garnish.

 ## gluten free
also dairy, egg & nut free

Follow the recipe on the left, but use a gluten-free bread roll and substitute gluten-free croûtons to garnish, if using.

WATCH OUT FOR chilli, as some people can't tolerate it. Omit if in any doubt.

Leek & butternut squash soup

Home-made soups, both delicious and nourishing, call for home-made stock, but if you don't have time, find a bouillon powder you can trust. I've gone to town with the toppings: herbs, seeds, bacon, and cream, but just one or two will turn a plain soup into something substantial or fancy. A tip for gluten-avoiders is to keep a store of gluten-free croûtons handy for soup and salad garnishes.

    egg, gluten & nut free

1 tbsp nut-free flavourless vegetable oil
1 good-sized butternut squash
2 tbsp butter
2 leeks, white parts only, finely chopped
1½ tsp curry powder
½ tsp ground cumin
1 litre (1¾ pints) chicken or vegetable stock
1 tsp molasses or dark brown sugar (optional)

salt and freshly ground black pepper to season
2 tbsp chopped fresh coriander or parsley
3 tbsp single cream

PREPARATION TIME 1¼ hours
COOKING TIME 20 minutes plus reheating
SERVES 8

dairy free
also egg, gluten & nut free

Follow the recipe on the left, but replace the butter with dairy-free spread and use soya cream alternative instead of the cream.

SERVING SUGGESTION Serve garnished with a swirl of double cream, chopped parsley or coriander, toasted squash seeds, or crumbled fried bacon (shown right).

WATCH OUT FOR stock cubes and bouillon. Check that they are dairy free or gluten free as necessary. Some people are sensitive to chilli, so omit the curry powder if need be.

1 Preheat the oven to 190°C (375°F, gas 5). Halve the butternut squash lengthways and scoop out the seeds. Brush the cut surfaces with the oil and bake face down on a baking sheet for 1 hour or until the flesh is soft. When cool enough to handle, scoop out the pulp and discard the skin.

2 Melt the butter in a heavy-based pan. Add the leeks and cook gently for about 3 minutes until softened, but not browned. Add the curry powder and cumin and cook for 1 minute.

3 Add the roasted squash, stock, and the molasses or sugar. Season lightly. Bring to the boil, reduce the heat, and cover and simmer for 20 minutes.

4 Purée the soup in a blender or food processor until there are no lumps. You may need to do this in two batches if it won't fit in your blender or food processor. Return to the saucepan. Stir in the chopped coriander or parsley and the cream. Taste and re-season, if necessary. Reheat but do not reboil. Ladle into warm soup bowls, season to taste with salt and pepper and garnish lavishly (see suggestion, right).

Pictured opposite ▶

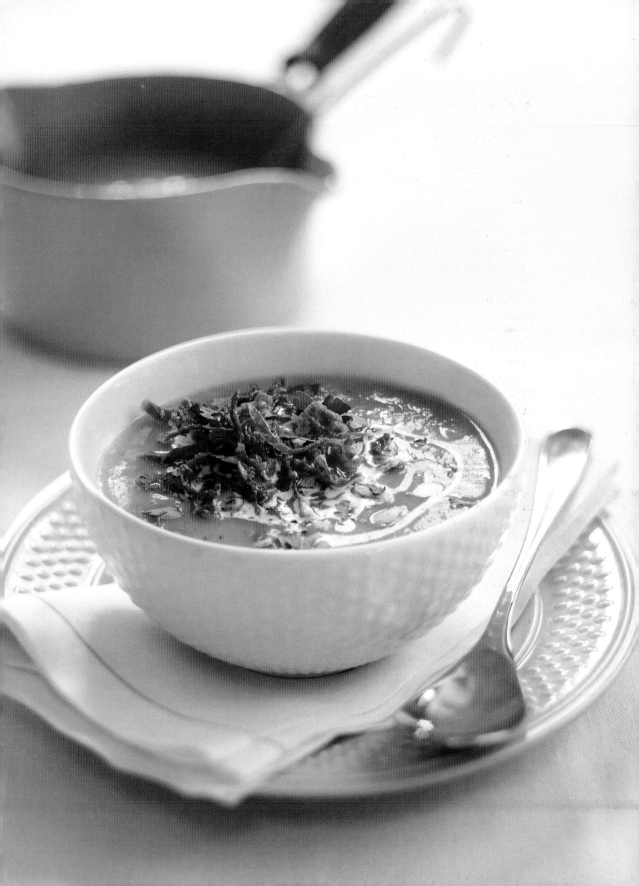

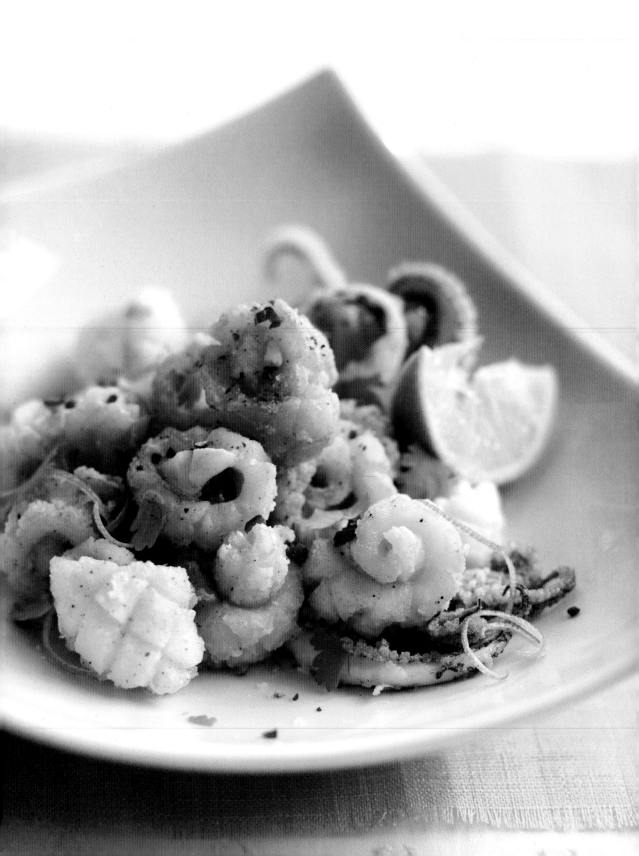

Crispy squid

If you thought you couldn't have light crispy fried food without egg or wheat, try this. It's inspired by the Chinese restaurant staple "salt and pepper squid", where seafood is rolled in seasoned cornflour and deep fried. Serve with sweet chilli sauce and lime wedges or Mayonnaise (p.210) with a dash of chilli sauce and lime juice stirred into it.

    dairy, egg, gluten & nut free

55g (2oz) cornflour
½ tsp chilli powder
½ tsp five-spice powder
½ tsp ground turmeric
½ tsp celery salt
salt and freshly ground black
 pepper to season
4 large squid, about 1kg (2¼lb),
 cleaned and slit open, and
 tentacles cut in short lengths
corn oil or other nut-free
 flavourless oil for frying

to garnish
roughly chopped fresh coriander
 leaves
finely chopped red pepper or red
 chillies, deseeded (if tolerated)
grated or pared zest of ½ lime
1 lime, cut into quarters

PREPARATION TIME 15 minutes
COOKING TIME 5 minutes
SERVES 4–6

WATCH OUT FOR chillies as some people cannot tolerate them. Omit the chilli powder and chilli garnish, if necessary. This dish is not suitable for people with a shellfish allergy.

TIP If you can't find large squid, buy baby squid – remove the tentacles and trim off the hard core at the base of them. Split and score each squid as in the recipe, but leave whole – they will curl beautifully when fried. Alternatively, if you can only buy squid rings, dust these in the cornflour mixture and fry in the same way.

1 Mix the cornflour with the chilli and five-spice powders, ground turmeric, and celery salt. Season with salt and pepper.
2 Wash the squid and pat them dry. Open out, score the inside surfaces lightly with a sharp knife in a cross-hatch pattern and cut the squid into 2.5cm (1in) pieces.
3 Heat the oil for deep-frying in a deep-fat fryer or wok to 190°C (375°F) or until a cube of day-old bread browns in 20 seconds.
4 Coat the squid pieces and the tentacles in the cornflour mixture and deep fry in batches for 45–60 seconds or until the squid pieces turn a light golden colour. A good rule of thumb is that the pieces are ready when the bubbling sound dies away. Be careful not to overcook or the squid will turn rubbery.
5 Drain on kitchen paper. Keep warm in a low oven until all the batches are fried. Pile the squid onto small warm dishes and garnish each with chopped coriander leaves, finely chopped red pepper or chillies, lime zest, and a wedge of lime.

SIDE DISHES, STARTERS & LIGHT MEALS

Fresh spring rolls

Basically a prawn, herb, and pork salad rolled in a soft rice paper wrapper, this is one of the most refreshing and elegant starters. Unlike most spring rolls it isn't deep-fried. A Vietnamese speciality, serve it with Vietnamese dipping sauce (p.210), Hoisin sauce, or even a peanut sauce (although you'll have to get a recipe elsewhere as I just couldn't include peanut sauce in an allergy friendly cookbook!).

    dairy, egg, gluten & nut free

rice paper wrappers (*banh trang*)
   20cm (8in) in diameter
4 large leaves of soft lettuce,
   each torn in half
30g (1oz) rice vermicelli, cooked
   according to packet
   instructions and drained
1 carrot, peeled and cut into
   julienne strips
115g (4oz) cooked pork (ideally
   pork belly), cut into thin strips
30g (1oz) bean sprouts

8 leaves of Thai basil (optional)
16–24 medium-sized cooked prawns
8 sprigs of coriander
8 leaves of mint

PREPARATION TIME 40 minutes
COOKING TIME 5 minutes for
   vermicelli
SERVES 4 as a starter (makes 8 rolls)

TIP The trick to wrapping rice papers is to do it when they have just reached the soft and pliable stage. Place the filling at the bottom of the wrapper and fold the sides in neatly. If you've not done it before, have a few spare to practise with first.

WATCH OUT FOR seafood. This dish is not suitable for people who are allergic to crustaceans. Omit the prawns and increase the pork or bean sprouts if necessary.

1 Have a large shallow bowl of warm water ready to soften the rice paper wrappers. Drop a wrapper into the water for 20 seconds and then place on kitchen paper.
2 Place half a lettuce leaf on the edge of the rice paper nearest to you. Put a tablespoon each of rice vermicelli and carrot strips on the lettuce and add a few strips of pork, several bean sprouts, and a Thai basil leaf, if using.
3 Bring up the nearest edge of the rice paper wrapper and roll it over the contents. Fold in the sides. You should now have the beginnings of a fairly tight cylinder.
4 Place 2–3 prawns in the crease between the rolled and unrolled portions of the rice paper and a sprig of coriander and a mint leaf next to the row of prawns. When fully rolled, the prawns and herbs will show through the translucent wrapper.
5 Now roll the rice paper into a cylinder. Place the roll, seam side down, on a large, flat plate to help seal it, and cover with a damp tea towel while you make the remaining spring rolls.
6 Serve immediately or store at room temperature, covered in cling film, for up to 2 hours.

Tabbouleh

This refreshing salad of parsley and tomatoes includes bulgur wheat – but the gluten-free version, using quinoa, has a slightly nutty flavour and is every bit as delicious. It is excellent as a starter or side dish.

   dairy, egg & nut free

55g (2oz) bulgur wheat
120ml (4fl oz) water
115g (4oz) chopped fresh parsley
15g (½oz) chopped fresh mint
1 small onion, chopped
4 spring onions, chopped
4 medium tomatoes, chopped

4 tbsp olive oil
4 tbsp lemon juice
salt and freshly ground black pepper

PREPARATION TIME 10 minutes
COOKING TIME 5–10 minutes
SERVES 4

1 Rinse the bulgur wheat in a sieve and drain. Bring the water to the boil, add the bulgur, bring back to the boil, reduce the heat and simmer gently until tender and the grain has absorbed the liquid, about 5–10 minutes.
2 Tip into a bowl and leave to cool.
3 Add the remaining ingredients, seasoning to taste with salt and pepper. Chill and serve on the day of making.

 gluten free
also dairy, egg & nut free

Follow the recipe on the left, but substitute quinoa for the bulgur wheat and cook in 150ml (5fl oz) of water. Cook for 5–10 minutes until all the liquid has been absorbed.

TIP In Lebanese restaurants, tabbouleh is sometimes served with lettuce leaves. Wrap a spoonful in a leaf and eat it with your fingers.

Cucumber & wakame salad

This light, fresh-tasting salad (pictured on page 100) is a perfect accompaniment to grilled fish and meats and is a version of a popular Japanese salad called *sunomono* (literally "things of vinegar").

    dairy, egg, gluten & nut free

15g (½oz) dried wakame seaweed
1 cucumber, peeled, deseeded, and diced
3 spring onions, sliced (optional)
for the dressing
2 tbsp rice vinegar
2 tsp mirin (rice wine)

2 tsp soy sauce
½ tsp clear honey

PREPARATION TIME 15 minutes
SERVES 4

1 Put the wakame in a bowl, cover with lukewarm water, and leave to soak for 10–15 minutes. Drain and trim away any rough stems, then cut the seaweed into strips. Place in a bowl with the cucumber and spring onions, if using.
2 Mix the dressing ingredients together until thoroughly blended and pour over the salad. Mix gently and serve immediately.

TIP Wakame, sometimes called sea vegetable, is seaweed sold in dried form in many Asian supermarkets and health food stores (see Resources, pp.218–219). When placed in water it softens to a glossy green vegetable that tastes and looks a little like spinach but needs no cooking.

SERVING SUGGESTIONS This is a delicious accompaniment to Miso marinated salmon (p.101).
Garnish with sesame seeds. If allergic to sesame seeds, a few pink pickled ginger slivers make an attractive alternative.

Middle Eastern salad

This simple salad is made special by the addition of two uniquely Middle Eastern ingredients. The bright pink pickled turnips get their colour from being pickled in beetroot juice and add tanginess to the salad. Deep red sumac powder is a popular seasoning made from the berries of the same name and has a pleasant lemony taste. If you have trouble finding it, just use paprika instead.

    dairy, egg, gluten & nut free

1 pink pickled turnip, drained
  and finely diced
1–1½ cucumbers, peeled,
  deseeded, and thinly sliced
2 medium tomatoes, finely
  diced or 8–10 cherry tomatoes,
  halved
1 spring onion, finely chopped
4 tbsp lemon juice
2 tbsp olive oil
powdered sumac or paprika to
  garnish (optional)

PREPARATION TIME 5 minutes
SERVES 4

1 Mix together the chopped vegetables.
2 Just before serving, dress with the oil and lemon juice and season with salt and pepper to taste. Sprinkle with powdered sumac or paprika and serve.

SERVING SUGGESTIONS Serve with dips such as Red pepper dip (p.211) or hummus and flatbreads as a starter, or as part of a main course with grilled lamb chops.

"Looks pretty in a glass bowl for a summer party or a girls' lunch"

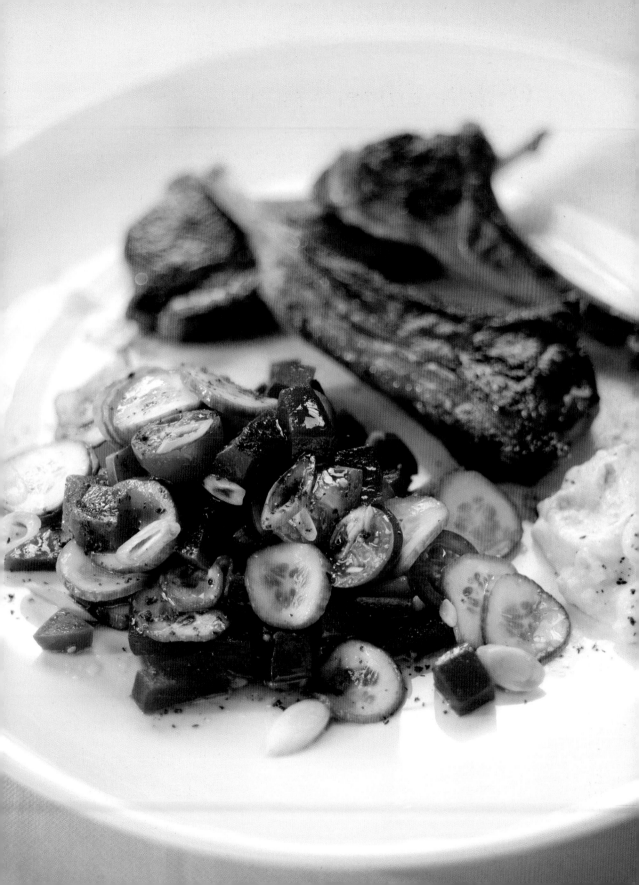

Gratin gallois

This version of the classic French *gratin dauphinois* is made near us in Wales. Unsurprisingly, it incorporates the national vegetable, leeks, and it is utterly delicious served bubbling hot. The vermouth brings out the flavours of the leeks, and the potatoes are deliciously crispy on top and creamy underneath. Serve with Honeyed Welsh lamb (p.132) or any roast or stew.

   egg, gluten & nut free

1½ tbsp flavourless nut-free oil, plus extra for greasing
450g (1lb) leeks, white parts only, finely chopped – yields around 340g (12oz)
600ml (1pint) single cream
1 bay leaf
2 tbsp dry vermouth
900g (2lb) floury potatoes, peeled and thinly sliced
2 garlic cloves, finely chopped
salt and freshly ground black pepper to season
freshly grated nutmeg to season

PREPARATION TIME 30 minutes
COOKING TIME 1¼ hours
SERVES 4–6

 dairy free
egg, gluten & nut free

Prepare as for the recipe on the left, but substitute an equal quantity of soya cream alternative for the whipping cream.

TIP Nutmeg is a fruit, not a nut, and therefore safe for people with nut allergies.

1 Preheat the oven to 180°C (350°F, gas 4). Grease a 1.2 litre (2 pint) gratin dish with oil.
2 In a heavy-based saucepan, fry the leeks in the oil until softened, but not coloured.
3 Add the cream, bay leaf and vermouth and simmer for 5 minutes.
4 Bring the cream mixture back to the boil and add the potatoes. Mix carefully with a large spoon to ensure the potatoes are evenly coated with the cream mixture.
5 Spoon half of the potato mixture into the gratin dish. Sprinkle over the garlic and season with salt and pepper. Add the remaining half of the potato mixture and season again with salt and pepper. Grate fresh nutmeg over the top.
6 Bake for about 1¼ hours or until brown and bubbling. The potatoes should be tender when a knife is inserted in the centre.

SIDE DISHES, STARTERS & LIGHT MEALS

Roast potatoes with garlic & sea salt

These are everything a roast potato should be – crisp, crunchy, and brown on the outside and fluffy on the inside. Don't just serve them with roasts – they work well with grills, braised dishes and stews, too. Ring the changes by sprinkling with herbs, such as rosemary or sage leaves, 20 minutes before the end of cooking or shake in a few drops of balsamic vinegar or pinches of paprika just before serving.

    dairy, egg, gluten & nut free

8 medium-sized potatoes, peeled and quartered
4 tbsp olive oil
1 head of garlic, separated into cloves
sea salt

PREPARATION TIME 8 minutes
COOKING TIME 30–40 minutes
SERVES 4–6

1 Preheat the oven to 220°C (425°F, gas 7).
2 Measure the oil into a large roasting tin and place in the oven to get hot.
3 Cook the potatoes in a pan of boiling water for 2 minutes. Drain and cool under cold water. Dry them well, using a tea cloth.
4 Carefully place the potatoes and unpeeled garlic cloves in the hot oil in the roasting tin. Turn them around to coat them evenly with the oil. Sprinkle with the sea salt and return to the oven.
5 Roast for 30–40 minutes until the potatoes are nicely browned with crispy edges. Turn the potatoes twice during cooking.

"Everyone loves them – it would be hard to imagine Sunday lunch without roast potatoes"

Fish pie

A winning combination of firm white fish and prawns in a creamy, parsley-flecked béchamel sauce under a mound of crispy-topped mashed potato, makes this a fabulous lunch or supper dish. You can vary the fish according to taste or season. Serve with buttered samphire, mixed peppery leaves, or a tomato salad to add contrasting flavour and colour.

  ## egg & nut free

750g (1lb 10oz) cod, halibut, or other white fish, filleted
250g (8½oz) smoked haddock or other smoked fish
500ml (16fl oz) milk
1 small onion, roughly chopped
bay leaf (optional)
100g (3½oz) butter
30g (1oz) plain flour
1.5kg (3lb 3oz) potatoes, peeled and quartered
2 tbsp single cream or milk

salt and freshly ground black pepper to season
225g (8oz) cooked peeled prawns
1 tbsp capers in brine, drained, rinsed, and chopped (optional)
2 tbsp chopped fresh parsley leaves
15g (½oz) Parmesan, grated (optional)

PREPARATION TIME 1¼ hours
COOKING TIME 45 minutes
SERVES 4–6

1 Preheat the oven to 190°C (375°F, gas 5).
2 Put the fish in a large saucepan, add the milk and poach the fish gently for 5 minutes; it should be slightly undercooked at this stage.
3 Transfer the fish to a plate with a draining spoon. When cool, remove the skin, cut the fish into large chunks and place in a 1.5 litre (2¾ pint) ovenproof dish.
4 Add the chopped onion and bay leaf (if using) to the fish milk. Bring to the boil. Remove from the heat and leave to stand for 10 minutes. Strain.
5 Make a white sauce by melting 45g (1½oz) of the butter in a saucepan and stirring in the flour. Cook, stirring for 1 minute. Whisk in the infused milk a little at a time, ensuring there are no lumps. When all the milk is incorporated, bring to the boil and cook for 2 minutes, whisking all the time. Remove from the heat.
6 Meanwhile, boil the potatoes for about 15 minutes or until cooked through. Mash with the remaining butter and the cream or milk and season with salt and pepper.
7 Add the prawns, capers, and parsley to the fish, season with salt and pepper, and pour over the white sauce. Top with the mashed potatoes and use a fork to rough up the surface to make it crispy when cooked. Dust with Parmesan cheese, if liked. Bake for 45 minutes until the top is crispy and golden.
Pictured opposite ▷

 ## dairy free
also egg & nut free

Follow the recipe on the left, but use dairy-free spread in place of butter; soya, rice, or oat milk instead of cow's milk; and soya cream alternative for single cream. Use dairy-free Parmesan.

 ## gluten free
also egg & nut free

Follow the recipe on the left, but for the white sauce, substitute gluten-free plain white flour or a half-and-half mix of rice flour and cornflour for the plain flour. You may need to increase the milk slightly to give a thick pouring sauce if using all gluten-free white flour.

WATCH OUT FOR fish and crustaceans. If allergic to crustaceans, but not white fish, omit the prawns and increase the fish to a total of 1.25kg (2¾lb).
 If you follow a gluten-free diet, make sure you buy capers in brine rather than malt vinegar.

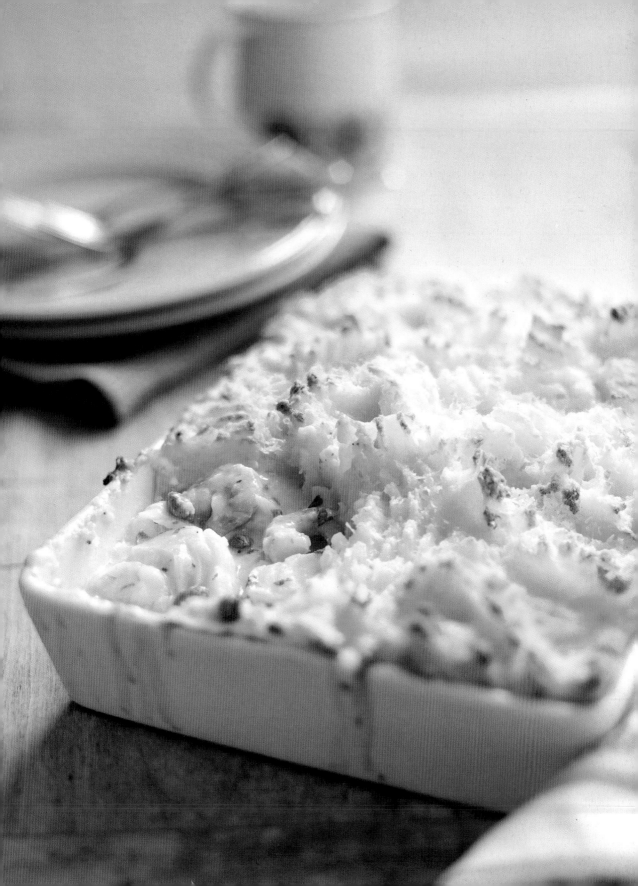

Tandoori fish

This quick-to-cook recipe makes an excellent light supper dish. In restaurants, red and yellow food colouring is used to achieve the brilliant orange colour of this famous Indian marinade, but I've made it optional, as the spices on their own give a mustardy-golden colour, which is just as attractive. Marinate for at least two hours to allow the subtle mixture of yogurt and spices to infuse the fish.

   egg, gluten & nut free

for the tandoori marinade
250ml (8½fl oz) plain yogurt
2 tbsp nut-free vegetable oil
2 garlic cloves, crushed
2 tsp grated fresh ginger
1 tsp garam masala
½ tsp ground turmeric
½ tsp chilli powder or paprika
salt to season
to finish
4 white fish fillets, about 225g
  (8oz) each, skinned if preferred

lemon or lime wedges (to garnish)
1 quantity of egg-, gluten-, and
  nut-free Raita (p.213)

PREPARATION TIME 5 minutes
  plus marinating time
COOKING TIME 15 minutes
SERVES 4

 dairy free
also egg, gluten & nut free

Follow the recipe on the left, but substitute soya yogurt for cow's milk yogurt in the marinade. Make the dairy-free Raita recipe on page 213.

SERVING SUGGESTION Serve with boiled plain or coconut rice and steamed green vegetables.

1 Mix all of the marinade ingredients together in a glass or other non-metallic bowl. Add the fish and coat thoroughly with the marinade.
2 Cover and chill for at least 2 hours or overnight.
3 Make the raita.
4 Preheat the oven to 220°C (425°F, gas 7). Remove the fish fillets from the marinade and drain off any excess. Place in an ovenproof dish and bake towards the top of the oven until the fish flakes easily with a fork, about 15 minutes. Transfer to warm plates. Garnish with lemon or lime wedges. Serve with the raita, a small side salad, and other accompaniments (see right).

WATCH OUT FOR chilli because some people cannot tolerate it – use paprika instead of chilli powder.

TIP If you decide to use red and yellow food dyes then add 1 teaspoon of yellow and 1½ teaspoons of red to the marinade. Make sure neither contain tartrazine, a known allergen.

FISH, MEAT & POULTRY

Marinated swordfish

This meaty fish suits Asian accents hence this fusion-style salsa verde. This makes a great dish for a barbecue as you can prepare the salsa in advance and the fish cooks in minutes. Keep an eye on it as it dries out quickly; it's best grilled or barbecued to medium. Serve the steaks with the salsa verde, lime wedges, and salads or noodles.

    dairy, egg, gluten, & nut free

2 x 450g (1lb) swordfish steaks,
  2.5–4cm (1–1¼in) thick,
  halved
for the marinade
2 tbsp gluten-free tamari or soy
  sauce
1 tbsp Thai fish sauce
1 tbsp sesame oil
1 small red onion, finely chopped
2 garlic cloves, finely chopped
2 tsp rice vinegar
2 tsp mirin (or dry sherry)
2 tbsp chopped fresh coriander
1 dried red chilli, crushed
flavourless nut-free oil for
  basting

for the Asian salsa verde
30g (1oz) fresh coriander leaves,
  roughly chopped
1½ tbsp grated fresh ginger
2 tbsp rice vinegar
2 tsp caster sugar
4 tbsp flavourless nut-free oil
6 spring onions, finely chopped
1 tsp lime juice
salt and freshly ground black pepper

PREPARATION TIME 10 minutes
  plus marinating time
COOKING TIME 8–10 minutes
SERVES 4

WATCH OUT FOR sesame oil; some people are allergic to sesame, in which case replace the oil with a flavourless nut-free oil. Make sure that the soy or tamari sauce is gluten free, if necessary.

TIP The steaks are also great barbecued. Place in a hinged wire rack and cook, 5–7.5cm (2–3in) from the coals. Cook for 4–5 minutes each side, brushing frequently with oil.

1 Mix the marinade ingredients together in a non-metallic or glass shallow bowl. Marinate the steaks for at least an hour, turning once or twice. Shake the marinade from the steaks before cooking.

2 Preheat the grill. Grill the fish, 10cm (4in) from the heat, for 4–5 minutes each side, until cooked through, brushing with oil occasionally.

3 For the Asian salsa verde, put the coriander, ginger, rice vinegar, sugar, and oil in a food processor and blend to a still-chunky, rough-textured paste, stopping and scraping down the sides as necessary. Stir in the chopped spring onions and the lime juice. Season to taste.

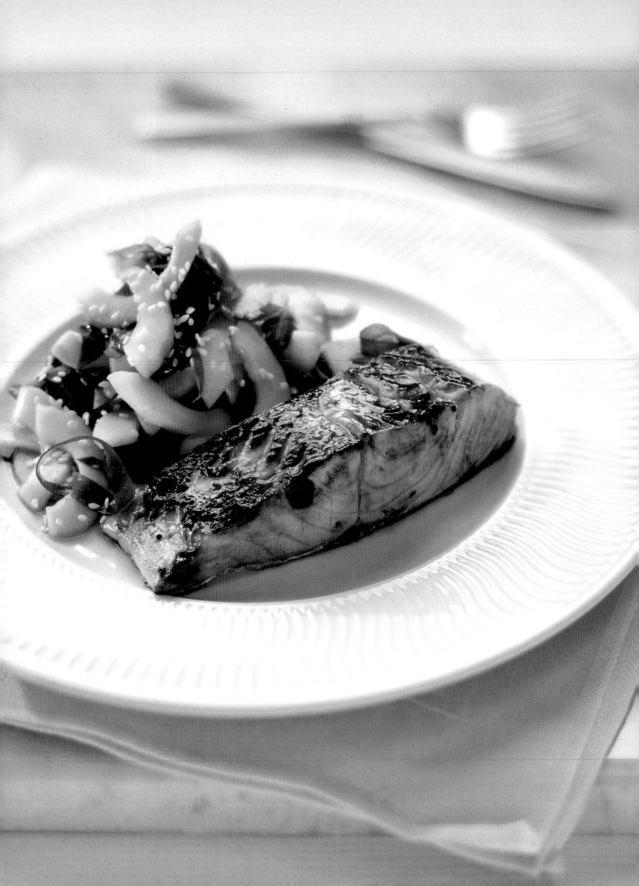

Miso marinated salmon

Marinating fish in miso and sake overnight is a traditional Japanese technique that works brilliantly with salmon. Miso, made from fermented soya beans, is a thick, salty paste with an underlying sharpness from the fermenting process and a rich caramel aftertaste that contributes well to the crisp browning of the fish. This easy dish is impressive enough for casual entertaining or a dinner party.

   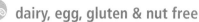 **dairy, egg, gluten & nut free**

3 tbsp mirin (rice wine)
2 tbsp sake
3 tbsp caster sugar
125g (4½oz) sweet rice miso paste
4 salmon fillets (with skin on), about 170g (6oz) each
Cucumber & wakame salad (p.91)

PREPARATION TIME 5 minutes plus cooling and marinating time
COOKING TIME 6 minutes
SERVES 4

1 For the sweet miso marinade, put the mirin and sake in a small saucepan. Add the sugar and heat gently, stirring until dissolved.
2 Bring to the boil, remove from the heat, and stir in the miso until thoroughly blended. Cool completely.
3 Place the salmon in a single layer in a non-metallic dish. Spoon over the marinade and turn the fish over to coat completely. Leave in the fridge to marinate for at least 4 hours or overnight.
4 When ready to serve, preheat the grill. Lay the fish, skin side up on foil on the grill rack. Grill for 3 minutes.
5 Turn the fish over and grill until lightly browned and the fish flakes easily with a fork, a further 3 minutes.
6 Serve with Cucumber & wakame salad (pictured right – see page 91 for recipe).

WATCH OUT FOR some varieties of miso that may include other grains, such as barley and wheat. Traditionally miso is made from fermented soya beans and koji, a fermented rice product, but check the ingredients before buying.

TIP If white miso paste (pale gold in colour) is difficult to get hold of, there are darker blends which work well in this recipe. However, avoid red miso (actually brown in colour) as this is by far the saltiest form.

SERVING SUGGESTION Good side dishes include rice, noodles (avoid egg or wheat-based noodles, if you can't tolerate them), spicy salad leaves, such as mizuna or watercress, and shredded daikon, turnip, or radishes. Sprinkle with black and white sesame seeds for stylish dinner party entertaining (if you can tolerate them).

Potato-crusted halibut

An unbelievably simple and effective recipe for halibut fillets with a crisp golden-brown potato topping and braised beetroot on the side. It's a recipe with mercifully little peeling involved and it works for all the "Big Four" allergies. Start the fish off in a frying pan and then transfer to the oven, where the beetroot is already cooking away.

    dairy, egg, gluten & nut free

for the braised beetroot
4 even-sized beetroot, about
  550g (1¼lb) in total, washed,
  but not trimmed or peeled
2 tbsp balsamic vinegar
for the halibut
4 thick halibut fillets, about
  200g (7oz) each, skinned if liked

salt and freshly ground black pepper
2 large potatoes, scrubbed, but
  not peeled
3 tbsp flavourless nut-free oil

PREPARATION TIME 20 minutes
COOKING TIME 1¼ hours
SERVES 4

SERVING SUGGESTION This is delicious served with lemony green beans. Steam green beans until just tender, about 6 minutes, and toss with olive oil, lemon zest, and juice.

1 Preheat the oven to 200°C (400°F, gas 6).

2 Wrap the beetroot individually in foil, sprinkling 1 tablespoon of water on each before sealing the foil.

3 Place on a baking sheet and cook for about 1 hour, or until the beetroot is tender all the way through. The peel slips off easily once they are cooked.

4 Top and tail the beetroot, cut into quarters and keep warm. Sprinkle with the balsamic vinegar just before serving and season with salt and pepper.

5 While the beetroot is cooking (after about 40 minutes), season the halibut fillets with salt and pepper.

6 Coarsely grate the potatoes and squeeze out as much excess water as possible. Pat the grated potatoes dry with kitchen paper.

7 Top each fillet with a thick, even layer of grated potato and press the topping down onto the fish.

8 Heat the oil in the frying pan until hot, almost smoking.

9 Using two spatulas or fish slices, one on the top of the fillet, one underneath, add the halibut fillets potato-side down to the pan. Push any stray potato back under the fish.

10 Fry until the potato crust is golden brown, about 5 minutes, then turn the fillets over carefully, again using both spatulas.

11 Place the frying pan in the oven if it is ovenproof. Otherwise, transfer the fillets to a roasting tin. Cook until the fillets are just cooked through, 8–10 minutes.

12 Transfer the fish and beetroot to warm serving plates. Serve with lemony green beans (see right).

Prawn dumplings

These little oriental morsels are filled with chopped prawns, spring onions, fresh ginger, and Thai fish sauce. They are cooked quickly in boiling water then served with a sweet chilli dipping sauce. They make an attractive starter for a dinner party or can be served for lunch or supper with a vegetable stir-fry. Tapioca flour is often used in Asian cookery and is gluten free.

   ## dairy, egg & nut free

for the dumplings
55g (2oz) plain flour plus extra
   for dusting
55g (2oz) tapioca flour
pinch of salt
120ml (4fl oz) warm water

for the filling
2 spring onions plus extra for
   garnish, if liked
200g (7oz) raw shelled king
   prawns, chopped
½ tsp grated fresh ginger
1 tsp Thai fish sauce

for the chilli dipping sauce
115g (4oz) granulated sugar
120ml (4fl oz) hot water
1 tsp crushed dried chillies
1 tbsp paprika
1 tsp grated fresh ginger
1 large garlic clove, crushed
1 tbsp Thai fish sauce
1–2 tbsp lime juice

PREPARATION TIME 30 minutes
   plus dough resting time
COOKING TIME 5 minutes
SERVES 4–6

 ## gluten free
also dairy, egg and nut free

Follow the recipe on the left, but substitute 55g (2oz) gluten-free plain white flour, plus extra for dusting, for the ordinary plain flour. Add 2 teaspoons of xanthan gum to the flours and use an extra 3–4 teaspoons of warm water to mix. There is no need to rest the dough before use.

WATCH OUT FOR chillies because some are sensitive to them.

SERVING SUGGESTION Garnish with spring onion curls. Trim 4 spring onions to about 7.5cm (3in) long from the white end. Make several cuts down the length of the white part, so they resemble tassels, then place in a bowl of iced water to make them curl.

TIPS If you prefer, use all plain flour instead of half tapioca flour.
   Check the consistency of the chilli dipping sauce and thin with a dash of cold water, if necessary.
   Use ready-made sweet chilli dipping sauce instead of the home-made, if you prefer. It is usually egg free, dairy free and gluten free, but check the label carefully as it may contain traces of nuts or sesame.

1 Sift the flours and salt into a bowl. Mix with the warm water to form a soft dough. Knead gently on a floured surface until smooth and elastic. Wrap in cling film and leave to rest for 30 minutes.

2 For the filling, finely chop the spring onions. Mix with the chopped prawns, ginger, and fish sauce.

3 Make the chilli sauce. Put the sugar in a saucepan with the water and heat, stirring, until melted. Stir in the remaining ingredients except the lime juice, bring to the boil and boil for 1 minute. Stir in the lime juice to taste. Tip into 4 small bowls and leave to cool.

4 On a floured surface, divide the dough into 24 balls and roll out to thin pancakes, about 6cm (2½in) in diameter. Loosen from the work surface, using a palette knife.

5 Put a spoonful of the filling on each pancake. Brush the edges with water. Fold over and pinch the edges together well.

6 Bring a large pan of water with a pinch of salt to the boil. Drop in the dumplings. Bring back to the boil, then simmer for 5 minutes, stirring gently to keep the dumplings separate. They will float to the surface as they cook.

7 Use a draining spoon to transfer to warm serving plates. Serve with a small pot of chilli dipping sauce on one side. Garnish with spring onion curls, if liked (see right).

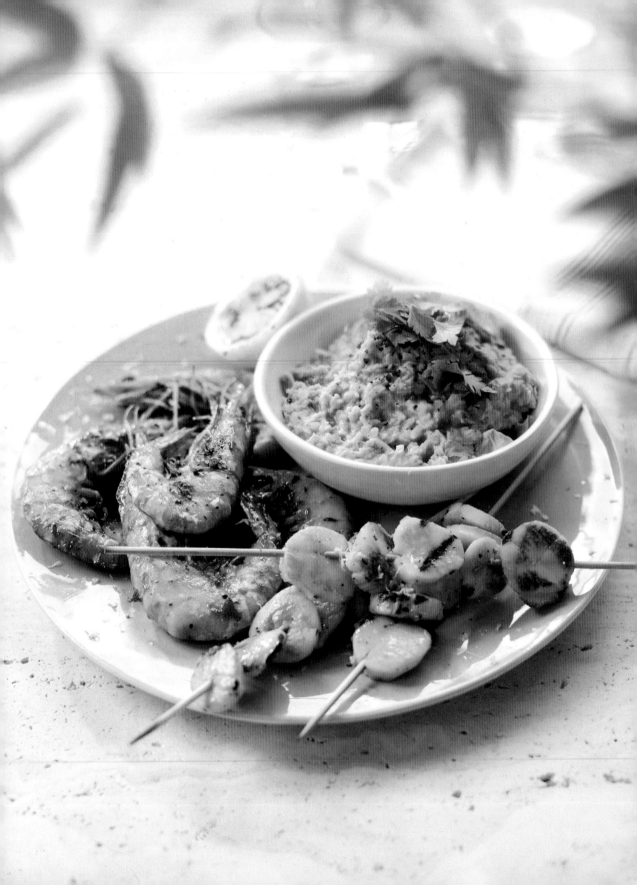

Scallops & prawns with lentils

An inspired pairing of aromatic simmered lentils with quick-cooked seafood that makes an excellent do-ahead dish with very little last minute effort. Influenced by the heady spice mix of red lentils in the Indian *masoor dhal*, the coral-coloured lentils turn a nice mustardy yellow when cooked. The dish works equally well with green, brown, or Puy lentils, though cooking times may vary.

   egg, gluten & nut free

12 large scallops without corals
12 jumbo prawns
3 tbsp sweet chilli sauce (optional)
3 tbsp lime juice (optional)
15g (½oz) butter
1 onion, finely chopped
2 garlic cloves
1 tbsp finely chopped fresh ginger
1 tsp ground cumin
1 tsp ground coriander
½ tsp chilli powder, cayenne, or paprika

200g (7oz) red lentils
1 litre (1¾ pints) water or stock
1 tbsp lime or lemon juice
2 tbsp double cream
salt and pepper to season
flavourless nut-free vegetable oil for grilling scallops
1 tsp finely chopped red chilli
2 tbsp fresh coriander leaves

PREPARATION TIME 10 minutes
COOKING TIME 30 minutes
SERVES 4

1 Pat the scallops dry on kitchen paper. Marinade the prawns in the chilli sauce and lime juice, if using.
2 Melt the butter in a saucepan and fry the onion, garlic, and ginger for 2 minutes, stirring, until softened. Add the cumin, coriander, and chilli powder, cayenne, or paprika to the mixture and fry for 1 minute, stirring.
3 Add the lentils and water or stock. Bring to the boil, then reduce to a simmer. Simmer for 25 minutes or until the lentils are soft but not mushy, stirring occasionally. Remove from the heat and stir in the lemon juice and cream and season well with salt and pepper. Place on a serving dish and keep warm.
4 Preheat the grill to medium.
5 Slice the scallops into two or three horizontally, depending on their size, and brush all over with oil.
6 Grill the prawns for about 2 minutes on each side, until pink. Grill the scallops for just 30 seconds each side or they will be over-cooked.
7 Scatter the chopped chilli and coriander leaves over the lentils. Serve immediately.
◀ **Pictured opposite**

 dairy free
also egg, gluten & nut free

Follow the recipe on the left, but substitute an equal quantity of soya or other dairy-free cream for the double cream used in the recipe.

TIP If barbecuing, place the prawns directly on the grill 10cm (4in) from the coals and cook for about 2 minutes each side. Skewer the scallops through the middle, brush with oil and grill 7.5cm (3in) from the coals for 30–60 seconds each side, turning once.

WATCH OUT FOR lentils – some pulses (lentils) are processed in factories that also process products containing gluten. Check for seafood allergies – prawns are crustacean, and scallops are molluscs. Some people cannot tolerate chillies – omit if in any doubt.

Chicken pie

A classic supper dish – ideal for family and guests. The vegetables are sautéed first for extra flavour and the chicken is lightly poached in stock and wine. Cornflour is used to make the sauce and the whole lot is combined under a crisp, glazed pastry crust. Even the egg-free version (pictured) has its own glaze, for a pie that looks as good as it tastes.

 ## nut free

2 tbsp flavourless nut-free
  vegetable oil
140g (5oz) button mushrooms
2 leeks, thinly sliced
600ml (1 pint) chicken stock
150ml (5fl oz) dry white wine
1 bay leaf
2 carrots, sliced
1kg (2¼lb) chicken fillets, cut
  into bite-sized pieces

3½ tbsp cornflour
salt and freshly ground black pepper
½ tsp chopped fresh thyme
1 quantity egg- and nut-free
  Shortcrust pastry (p.180)
1 egg, beaten

PREPARATION TIME 40 minutes
COOKING TIME 40 minutes
SERVES 6

1 Preheat the oven to 200°C (400°F, gas 6).
2 Heat the oil in a saucepan, add the mushrooms, and fry for 5 minutes. Remove the mushrooms to a plate. Add the leeks to the pan and fry for 2 minutes, stirring, and remove to a plate.
3 Add the stock, wine, bay leaf, and carrots to the pan, bring to the boil, reduce the heat and simmer for a further 5 minutes. Add the chicken and cook gently for a further 5 minutes. Remove the chicken and carrots to a plate.
4 In a small bowl, blend the cornflour with 4 tablespoons of the stock mixture and stir until smooth. Pour into the pan and cook, stirring, for 3 minutes until thickened. Season and remove from the heat.
5 Spoon the chicken, all the vegetables and the sauce into a deep 1.7 litre (3pt) pie dish. Stir in the thyme.
6 Roll out the pastry on a floured surface to 5mm (¼in) thick. Cut a pastry lid. Roll out the trimmings and cut a 1cm (½in) strip, long enough to go round the rim of the dish.
7 Dampen the edge of the pie dish with water and press the strip of pastry around the rim. Dampen the strip.
8 Carefully lift the pastry lid and place over the top of the pie dish and firmly press it to the strip all around to seal. Crimp or flute the edges together if you like. Make a small slit in the centre of the pastry to allow steam to escape. Glaze the pastry with beaten egg.
9 Bake until golden and the pie is hot through, about 40 minutes.

WATCH OUT FOR stock cubes, which may contain traces of dairy or gluten.

 ## dairy free
also nut free

Follow the recipe on the left, using one quantity of dairy-free Shortcrust pastry (p.180).

 ## egg free
also nut free

Follow the recipe on the left. To glaze, replace the egg with 2 tablespoons of milk or, if a shinier glaze is preferred, use the following gelatine glaze. Put 2 tablespoons of water in a small bowl and sprinkle over 1 tablespoon of gelatine. Leave to soften for 5 minutes then stand the bowl in a pan of gently simmering water and stir until dissolved completely. Brush over the pastry using a pastry brush, taking care not to let puddles of the glaze collect in the pastry hollows or crimped edges. **Pictured opposite** ▷

 ## gluten free
also nut free

Prepare as for the recipe on the left, using one quantity of gluten-free Shortcrust pastry (p.182). The gluten-free pie crust will have a slight yellowish hue because of the maize meal in the pastry.

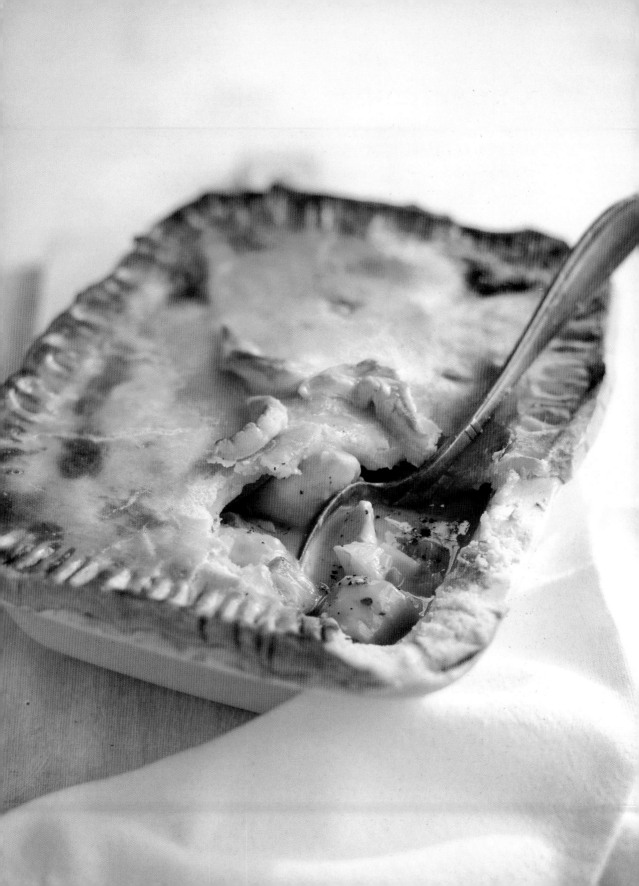

Chicken, olive & chickpea stew

A dish with characteristically North African flavours; sweet spices, chickpeas, lemon, and green olives meld together to make a meltingly delicious stew. It is easy to make and ideal for summer or winter eating. Serve with plenty of rice to soak up the juices. Alternatively, use couscous, either the real thing, or the quinoa version (see gluten-free recipe, p.135), or Basmati & wild rice pilaf (p.144).

    dairy, egg, gluten & nut free

4 tbsp light olive oil
4 chicken breasts on the bone, with skin on
1 onion, chopped
2 garlic cloves, crushed
1 tsp ground cumin
2 tsp ground turmeric
½ tsp coriander seeds, crushed
4 cardamom pods, lightly crushed
240ml (8fl oz) chicken stock
juice of 1 lemon

1 x 425g (15oz) can of chickpeas, drained and rinsed
12 pitted green olives, soaked in water for 2 hours if salty
salt and freshly ground black pepper

PREPARATION TIME 12 minutes
COOKING TIME 40–50 minutes
SERVES 4

1 Heat 2 tablespoons of the oil in a large flameproof casserole dish and brown the chicken pieces on both sides. Remove with a draining spoon and set aside.
2 Heat the remaining oil and sauté the onions and garlic for 2 minutes until softened but not browned. Stir in the cumin, turmeric, coriander, and cardamom and cook gently for 1 minute. Stir in the stock, lemon juice, and chickpeas.
3 Bring to the boil, reduce the heat, cover and simmer for 40–50 minutes or until the chicken is tender. Add the olives 10 minutes before the end of cooking.
4 Season with salt and pepper just before serving.

WATCH OUT FOR stock cubes, which may contain traces of dairy or gluten, if you're cooking for people with severe dairy or gluten sensitivities.

VARIATION If you like a lemony taste, add the squeezed lemon halves into the stew and remove just before serving.

"This one-pot supper dish releases its wonderful fragrances as soon as you lift the lid"

Lemon thyme grilled chicken

Delicious, versatile, and quick, this herbed, lemon-scented grilled chicken is perfect for any meal. If you can, buy chicken pieces with the bone still in as it contributes to the flavour, and keep the skin on as it crisps beautifully as it cooks. Noodles or boiled rice are a perfect match – all you need is a well flavoured salad to accompany it.

    dairy, egg, gluten & nut free

8 chicken thighs or drumsticks or
  4 chicken breasts on the bone,
  with skin on
juice of 1 lemon
1 garlic clove, crushed
2 tsp fresh thyme leaves
½ tsp finely chopped fresh
  rosemary
4 tbsp olive oil
salt and pepper to season
finely grated zest of 1 lemon

PREPARATION TIME 5 minutes
  plus marinating
COOKING TIME 18–20 minutes
  (grilled), 30 minutes (roasted)
SERVES 4

SERVING SUGGESTION Serve with a salad of chopped tomatoes, chickpeas, and finely sliced red onions dressed with olive oil and wine vinegar, or mixed salad leaves with a honey and mustard dressing.

1 Mix the lemon juice (reserve the squeezed lemon halves for later), garlic, herbs, 2 tablespoons of the oil, and a little salt and pepper in a shallow non-metallic bowl and marinate the chicken pieces for at least an hour.

2 Preheat the grill to moderate. Grill the chicken pieces, skin side down, 10cm (4in) from the heat for 10 minutes, then turn over. Brush with any remaining marinade and grill until cooked through, a further 8–10 minutes. Alternatively, roast the chicken pieces in the oven at 190°C (375°F, gas 5) for about 30 minutes. Tuck the squeezed lemon halves into the roasting tin for added flavour.

4 Transfer to warm serving plates and spoon any pan juices over. Garnish with the lemon zest before serving.

VARIATION Replace the thyme and rosemary with a handful of torn fresh basil leaves, scattered over the chicken 10 minutes before the end of the cooking time.

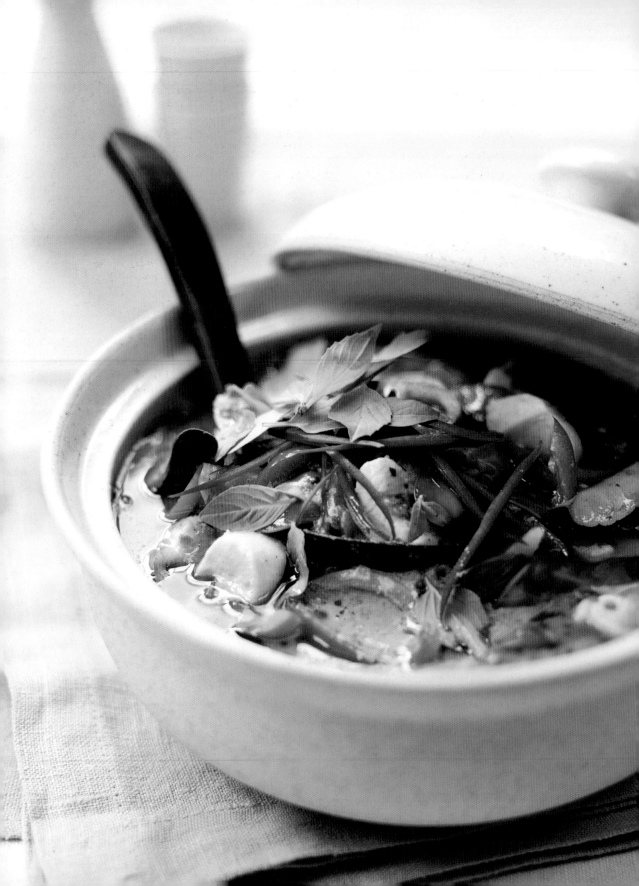

Thai green chicken curry

A virtually authentic Thai curry with the characteristic aroma and flavour of coconut, fish sauce, ginger, curry, and herbs. I've substituted colourful red and yellow peppers for the more traditional pea aubergines used in Thailand. This version has plenty of kick from the green curry paste and the shredded red chilli, but for those who like more firepower, there are optional green chillies.

    dairy, egg, gluten & nut free

2 x 400ml (14fl oz) cans of coconut milk

450g (1lb) skinless chicken breasts, cut into 2.5cm (1in) pieces

4 kaffir lime leaves, 2 left whole and 2 finely shredded

a little nut-free vegetable oil

2–3 red, orange, or yellow peppers, sliced (optional)

2 tbsp Thai green curry paste

3 tbsp Thai fish sauce

2 tsp palm sugar or brown sugar

3–4 green chillies, deseeded and crushed (optional)

2.5cm (1in) piece galangal (*kha*) peeled and shredded

150g (5½oz) mangetout (optional)

1 red chilli, deseeded and finely shredded

10–12 Thai sweet basil leaves, torn

PREPARATION TIME 10 minutes
COOKING TIME 20 minutes
SERVES 4

TIPS If you can't get galangal (a root that resembles ginger), just use a 1cm (½in) piece of fresh ginger. Grated zest of ½ lime is a good substitute for the lime leaves.

If you don't like your curries too hot, replace the shredded red chilli with a quarter of a red (bell) pepper, deseeded and thinly sliced.

WATCH OUT FOR chilli, as some people can't tolerate it. Omit if need be.

1 Open both cans of coconut milk and spoon the thick coconut cream that has risen to the top of the cans into a saucepan. Pour the thinner milk at the bottom of the cans into a measuring jug for use later.

2 Add the chicken and the 2 whole kaffir lime leaves to the thick coconut cream. Cook on a moderately high heat for 10 minutes or until the chicken is just cooked through. Remove the chicken to a plate using a draining spoon.

3 Boil the coconut cream until it thickens and the oil separates out. It will look curdled at this stage but don't worry. It will be used to thicken and flavour the sauce (in step 5).

4 In a large frying pan, fry the peppers (if using) in oil for about 3 minutes. Set aside. Fry the curry paste in a tablespoon of the remaining coconut milk for 1–2 minutes until the fragrance is released. Add the fish sauce and sugar and stir.

5 Add the remaining coconut milk, green chillies (if using), galangal, and mangetout (if using). Stir and cook on a moderate heat for 5 minutes. Return the peppers (if using), chicken, and coconut cream to the pan and cook for about 5 minutes to make sure that the chicken is heated through. Scatter the shredded kaffir lime leaves, red chilli, and sweet basil leaves over the curry just before you've finished heating through the meat.

6 Serve immediately with steamed or boiled rice.

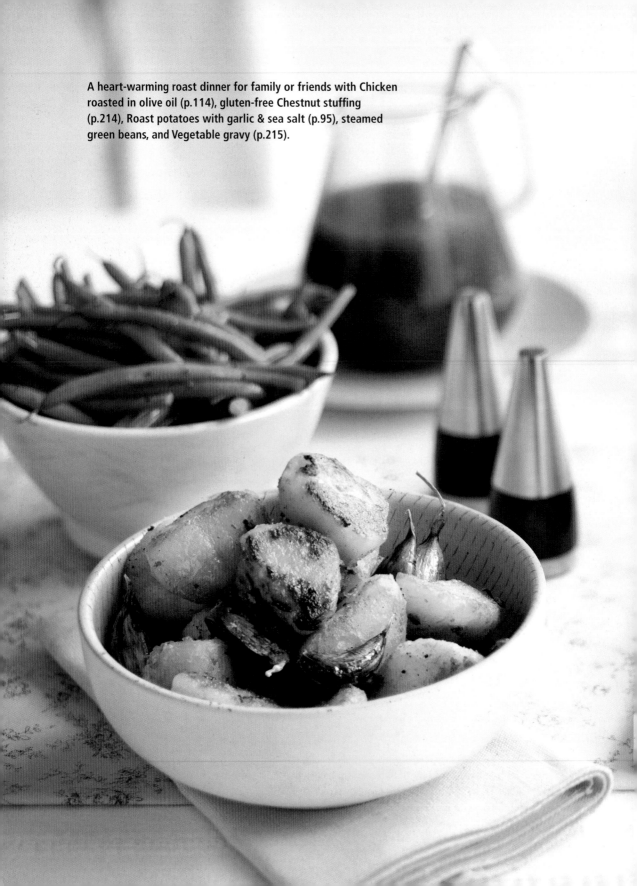

A heart-warming roast dinner for family or friends with Chicken roasted in olive oil (p.114), gluten-free Chestnut stuffing (p.214), Roast potatoes with garlic & sea salt (p.95), steamed green beans, and Vegetable gravy (p.215).

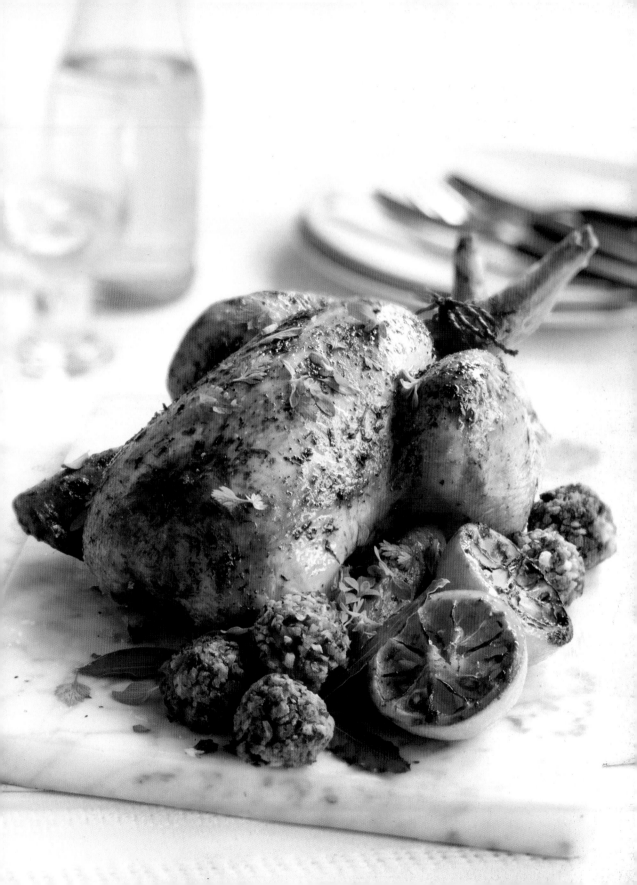

Chicken roasted in olive oil

Everyone has their own recipe for chicken or other celebratory birds. This one is delicious and has the benefit of being naturally dairy free. If you are making a family meal or festive roast chicken or turkey, accompany it with Vegetable gravy (p.215), Roast potatoes with garlic & sea salt (p.95), lightly steamed green beans, and Chestnut stuffing (p.214).

    dairy, egg, gluten & nut free

1.1–1.4kg (2½–3lb) free-range chicken
1 lemon
1 onion, halved
fresh parsley, chervil, or marjoram
4 tbsp olive oil
salt and freshly ground black pepper

PREPARATION TIME 5 minutes
COOKING TIME 1 hour
SERVES 4

1 Preheat the oven to 220°C (425°F, gas 7).
2 Cut the lemon in half and squeeze the juice over the chicken. Place the squeezed lemon halves in the cavity along with the onion halves. Alternatively, for an attractive garnish, place the lemon halves in the roasting tin alongside the bird.
3 Finely chop the herbs and mix them with a little olive oil. Gently prise the skin away from the chicken breast and use the herbs to stuff the gap between the skin and the chicken breast.
4 Using your hands, rub olive oil into the skin of the chicken and then season generously with salt and pepper.
5 Cook for 1 hour or until the chicken is browned and the juices run clear when a skewer is inserted into the thigh.
◀ **Pictured on previous page**

"This has crispy golden skin, soft white meat, and a hint of lemon in the juices"

Duck with apples & celeriac

Not just fabulous to eat, this special occasion duck is served on a bed of sautéed apple and celeriac with a delicious deep-red wine, and fig gravy. Its beautiful autumnal colours make it a feast for the eyes, too. Cooking the duck is an easy stove-top recipe, and if you make the gravy ahead of time, the whole dish can be assembled in about 20 minutes.

   egg, gluten & nut free

for the gravy
240ml (8fl oz) red wine
120ml (4fl oz) well-flavoured
  duck or chicken stock
1 sprig thyme or 1 bouquet garni
1 onion, quartered
5cm (2in) piece of orange peel
4 dried figs, halved
for the duck
2 large eating apples

700g (1lb 6oz) celeriac
1 tbsp wine or cider vinegar
30g (1oz) butter
4 medium-sized duck breasts, skin on

PREPARATION TIME 25 minutes
COOKING TIME 50 minutes
SERVES 4

1 Place the gravy ingredients in a saucepan and bring them to the boil. Reduce to a simmer and simmer very low for 30 mins or until the figs are soft. Discard the onion, thyme sprig (or bouquet garni), and orange peel. Put the figs and a minimal amount of the liquid (6–8 tablespoons) in a food processor and blend until smooth. Mix the blended figs back into the gravy and set aside.

2 Peel and chop the apples into 1cm (½in) pieces. Peel and chop the celeriac into 1cm (½in) pieces and cover with water acidulated with wine or cider vinegar to prevent discoloration.

3 Steam the celeriac pieces for 3–5 minutes until just tender.

4 Brown the apple pieces in the butter until golden but still firm.

5 On a medium heat in a large frying pan, place the duck breasts skin-side down. When the fat begins to run, turn the heat up to medium-high for about 5 minutes. When the skins are brown, turn the breasts over and cook for 10–12 minutes, depending on how pink you like your duck. Cover the pan if it spatters. Use a slotted spoon to remove the duck and keep it warm.

6 Pour away the excess fat and add the gravy to the pan, scraping to incorporate any residues. Allow the gravy to bubble and reduce for 1–2 minutes. Season, remove from the heat, and keep warm.

7 Add the celeriac to the frying pan with the apples. Sauté them together briefly to warm through.

8 Slice each duck breast into thin slices. Tip the celeriac and apple mixture onto a warmed serving dish and top with the duck slices. Surround with gravy and serve immediately.

 dairy free
also egg, gluten & nut free

Follow the recipe on the left. In step 3, replace the butter with 2 tablespoons of light olive oil.

TIP If you want to make this dish look really professional, arrange vegetables on individual warmed plates, then slice the duck breast in 5mm (¼in) slices, and fan out over the vegetables. Pour red wine and fig gravy around the perimeter of the vegetables in a crescent.

VARIATION For a truly plutocratic touch, finely chop 50g (1¾oz) of duck foie gras and stir into the apple and celeriac at the end of step 7 just before removing from the heat.

WATCH OUT FOR foie gras, if using, as some has added butter. Check your stock cubes because some may contain traces of gluten or dairy.

FISH, MEAT & POULTRY

Fegato alla Veneziana

One of the best versions of liver and onions there is, this is also an easy, near-instant supper dish. The pre-preparation of frying the onions is simple and the finished dish only takes a couple of minutes. The vinegar is essential so don't leave it out. Serve with Grilled polenta (p.81), as they do in Venice, or with puréed potatoes and wilted spinach leaves, or braised *cavolo nero* (Italian cabbage).

   egg, gluten & nut free

2 tbsp light olive oil
2 mild onions, thinly sliced
8–12 very thin slices of calves
   liver, trimmed and cleaned
   (450g/1lb in total)
sea salt and freshly ground black
   pepper to season
45g (1½oz) butter
2 tbsp red wine vinegar

to garnish
chopped fresh parsley or sage

PREPARATION TIME 5 minutes
COOKING TIME 12 minutes
SERVES 4

 dairy free
also egg, gluten & nut free

Follow the recipe on the left, but use 2½ tablespoons of light olive oil rather than butter in step 3.

1 Heat the olive oil in a large frying pan over a moderate heat. Fry the onions, stirring frequently, until they are soft and golden brown, but not scorched, 8–10 minutes. Remove the onions from the pan with a draining spoon and set aside on a warmed plate.
2 Season the liver slices with sea salt and freshly ground pepper.
3 Increase the heat to medium high and add the butter. When the butter is foaming, add the seasoned liver slices and brown them, preferably in batches to avoid overcrowding. The hot pan sears the liver quickly, so you should need no more than 15 seconds for each side.
4 Return the onions to the side of the pan and toss briefly to heat through. Sprinkle the wine vinegar over, which will hiss and reduce quickly to a mere trace of liquid.
5 Transfer to warm plates, spooning over any pan juices and sprinkle with parsley or sage.

WATCH OUT FOR vinegars – please don't substitute grain-based or malt vinegars for red wine vinegar. It won't taste right and gluten-sensitives can't tolerate grain or malt vinegars.

Ragu Bolognese

Delicious with spaghetti, this ragu works well with any pasta, which has plenty of surface area for the sauce to cling to. It's a winner with corn pasta, too. Simmer it slowly and add the cream near the end, to make it as authentically Bolognese as possible. The best cheese to serve it with is Parmesan, and there are some pretty good dairy-free versions around now, too.

   ## egg, gluten, & nut free

2 tbsp olive oil
1 onion, finely chopped
2 garlic cloves, finely chopped
1 carrot, finely chopped
55g (2oz) bacon, pancetta, or prosciutto, chopped into 2cm (³⁄₄in) pieces
300g (10½oz) lean beef, minced
100g (3½oz) chicken livers, trimmed and chopped
150ml (5fl oz) dry white wine
400g (14oz) can of chopped tomatoes with their juice
2 tbsp tomato purée

sea salt and freshly ground black pepper to season
¼ tsp freshly grated nutmeg
1 bay leaf
4 tbsp double or whipping cream
chopped fresh parsley for garnishing (optional)

to serve
pasta of your choice
freshly grated Parmesan

PREPARATION TIME 20 minutes
COOKING TIME 2 hours
SERVES 4

 ## dairy free
also egg, gluten & nut free

Follow the recipe on the left, but use soya cream alternative instead of double or whipping cream and non-dairy Parmesan alternative (sometimes called vegan Parmesan) – beware as this can be quite salty.

1 Heat 1 tablespoon of oil in a flameproof casserole dish or heavy-based saucepan. Fry the onions for 2 minutes or until lightly golden. Add the garlic and carrot and fry for another 2 minutes. Add the bacon and cook for a further 2 minutes. Remove from the pan with a draining spoon and set aside.

2 Heat the remaining oil and fry the meat until browned, stirring all the time to break up the lumps. Add the chicken livers and mix in well. Return the vegetable and bacon mixture to the pan and combine with the beef and liver.

3 Add the wine, tomatoes, and tomato purée. Season with salt and pepper and add the grated nutmeg and bay leaf.

4 Bring to the boil, stirring, then reduce to as low as possible and simmer very gently until rich and tender for 1¼ hours, stirring occasionally. Stir in the cream and continue to simmer very gently for a further 45 minutes.

5 Serve the ragu stirred into pasta, with parsley, if liked, and a bowl of grated Parmesan.

Osso buco

This meltingly tender, rich, slow-simmered dish is a real treat. I didn't think the famous veal stew could be improved upon until I found an Italian recipe that suggested incorporating finely chopped carrots and celery into the rich tomato and wine sauce. Add the gremolata seasoning of parsley, lemon zest, and garlic right at the end for a wonderful, fresh and tangy contrast.

    dairy, egg, gluten & nut free

2 tbsp nut-free vegetable oi
4 large pieces of shin of veal (*ossi bucchi*), each at least 5cm (2in) thick
2 carrots, very finely chopped
1 celery heart, very finely chopped
250ml (8½fl oz) very dry white wine
400g (14oz) tomatoes, skinned and chopped (or 400g/14oz can of chopped tomatoes)

1 tbsp tomato purée
salt and freshly ground black pepper
for the gremolata
grated zest of 1 lemon
2 tbsp finely chopped fresh parsley
1 garlic clove, finely chopped

PREPARATION TIME 15 minutes
COOKING TIME 1½–2 hours
SERVES 4

SERVING SUGGESTION Serve with saffron-scented Risotto alla Milanese (pictured right – see page 145 for the recipe).

Dig out the marrow from the marrowbones and stir into the risotto.

TIP You can add a pinch of caster sugar with the tomatoes to bring out their flavour.

1 Heat the oil in a frying pan and lightly brown the veal pieces on both sides. Remove from the frying pan with a draining spoon and set aside.
2 Gently fry the chopped carrots and celery in the pan for about 2 minutes, stirring, until softened, but do not allow them to brown.
3 Transfer the vegetables to a flameproof casserole dish that is just large enough to fit the veal in a single layer (this keeps the liquid ingredients to the minimum and avoids a thinner sauce). Arrange the veal on top.
4 In a bowl, combine the wine, tomatoes, and tomato purée and season with salt and pepper. Pour the mixture over the meat and vegetables – it should just cover the meat. If necessary, top up with wine.
5 Bring to the boil and then reduce the heat to the barest simmer. Cover and cook gently for 1½–2 hours, removing the cover after the first hour. The stew is cooked when the meat is tender and loosening from the bones and the sauce is slightly reduced. Taste and re-season if necessary.
6 Just before serving, mix together the lemon zest, parsley, and garlic to make the gremolata and sprinkle it over the meat.

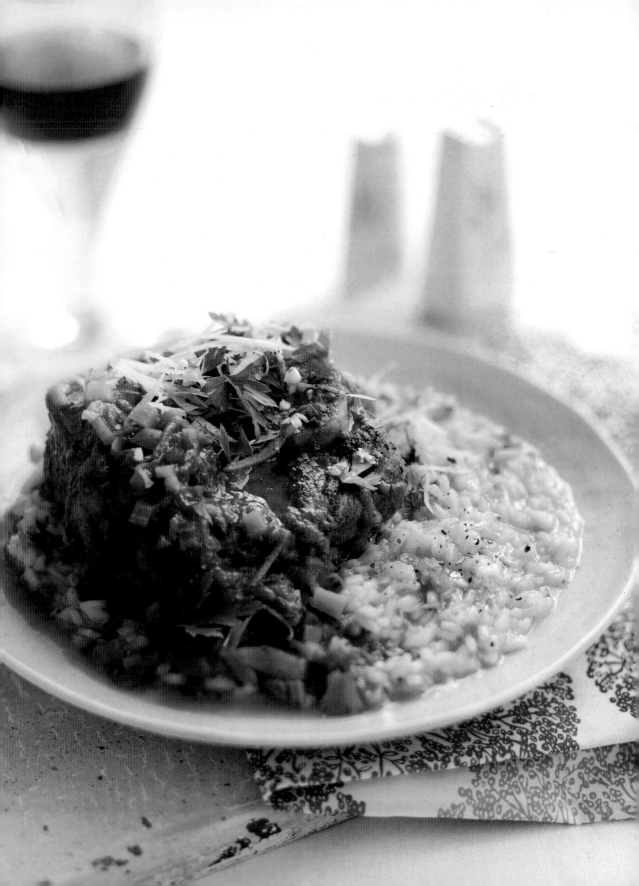

Vitello tonnato

An elegant, classic dish for hot summer days. The slices of cold roast veal in a creamy tuna-mayonnaise sauce need no more than boiled rice or new potatoes and a green salad to accompany them. A favourite for buffet lunches, Vitello tonnato looks at its most decorative arranged as overlapping slices with the sauce poured over and then decorated with capers and thinly sliced lemon.

   dairy, gluten, & nut free

3 tbsp olive oil
675g (1½lb) piece of boned
  veal loin
1 onion, quartered
1 carrot, chopped
1 celery stick, chopped
75ml (2½fl oz) dry white wine
75ml (2½fl oz) stock
1 bay leaf
salt and freshly ground black
  pepper
for the sauce
200g (7oz) drained, best quality
  canned tuna in oil
2 tbsp lemon juice
3 anchovy fillets, chopped

1 tbsp capers in brine plus extra
  to garnish
salt and freshly ground black pepper
125g (4½oz) shop bought mayonnaise
  or 1 quantity of Mayonnaise (p.210)
  or a ¼ quantity of Aïoli (p.209)
juices from the roast (to thin the sauce)
to garnish
½ lemon, thinly sliced (optional)
fresh parsley, roughly chopped
  (optional)

PREPARATION TIME 15 minutes
  plus chilling time
COOKING TIME 1 hour
SERVES 4

 egg free
also dairy, gluten & nut free

Follow the recipe on the left, but use shop-bought egg-free mayonnaise or 1 quantity of egg-free Mayonnaise (p.210) or a ¼ quantity of Aïoli (p.209).

TIPS Buy topside or shoulder of veal loin, in preference.
  If making in advance, slice and marinate the veal in a third of the sauce overnight for extra flavour.

1 Preheat the oven to 180°C (350°F, gas 4). Heat the oil in a frying pan and brown the joint quickly on all sides.
2 Spread the onion, carrot, and celery out in a large casserole dish and place the browned meat on top.
3 Add the wine, stock, bay leaf, and a little salt and pepper. Cover with the lid and roast in the oven for 1 hour, until tender, basting once or twice. Remove from the oven and leave to cool in the liquid. When cold, wrap the veal in foil, and chill until ready to serve. Strain the liquid and discard the vegetables, but reserve the liquid for thinning the sauce.
4 Make the sauce. In a food processor, blend together the tuna, lemon juice, anchovies, and capers to a smooth purée. Season to taste. Fold in the mayonnaise or aïoli, using 5–6 tablespoons of the reserved juices from the roast to thin the sauce to the consistency of thick cream.
5 Remove the veal from the fridge and allow it to come to room temperature. Arrange slices attractively on a serving dish. Pour over the sauce and decorate with thin slices of lemon and some scattered capers and fresh parsley, if liked.

Meatloaf

This is a great family meatloaf, crusty on top and juicily meaty underneath. It is comforting, nostalgic eating, especially when combined with mashed potatoes and Vegetable gravy (p.215). It's delicious, too, with a fresh tomato sauce or a big dollop of ketchup. I've suggested some additions but I'm sure you'll have your own. Enjoy the leftovers in sandwiches or cold with a green salad or coleslaw.

  ### dairy & nut free

1 tbsp nut-free vegetable oil plus extra for greasing
1 onion, chopped
450g (1lb) minced beef
225g (8oz) minced pork or sausage meat
1 tbsp Worcestershire sauce (optional)
2 garlic cloves, crushed
85g (3oz) breadcrumbs
1 tsp chopped fresh thyme leaves or ½ tsp dried
6 tbsp chopped fresh parsley

3 tbsp tomato ketchup
3 tbsp passata
salt and freshly ground black pepper to season
1 egg, beaten

PREPARATION TIME 10 minutes
COOKING TIME 1–1¼ hours
SERVES 4–6

1 Preheat the oven to 180°C (350°F, gas 4). For a soft-sided loaf that is crusty on top, line a 23 x 16cm (9 x 15in/2lb) loaf tin with baking parchment. If you prefer to hand mould the meatloaf, so that it will be crusty all the way around, line a baking sheet instead.
2 Fry the onion in the oil for 4 minutes, until softened and golden.
3 In a bowl, mix the meat, fried onions, Worcestershire sauce, if using, garlic, breadcrumbs, herbs, ketchup, and passata. Season well. Stir in the beaten egg to bind.
4 Transfer the mixture to the prepared tin or shape into a loaf roughly 23 x 16cm (9 x 5in) on the baking sheet.
5 Bake in the oven for 1–1¼ hours until browned on top and the sides are beginning to shrink away from the tin.
6 Turn out onto a warm plate. Pour any juices in the tin over the loaf. Slice and serve with mashed potatoes and gravy.

WATCH OUT FOR tomato ketchup, as it may contain traces of wheat or dairy, so check the labels carefully. Make sure the Worcestershire sauce is gluten free, if need be.

 ### egg free
also dairy & nut free

Follow the recipe on the left, but substitute 1 tablespoon of potato flour mixed with 2 tablespoons of water in place of the beaten egg and stir into the mixture in step 3.

 ### gluten free
also dairy & nut free

Follow the recipe on the left, but use gluten-free breadcrumbs. If using sausage meat rather than minced pork, ensure that no fillers that contain gluten have been added to the meat.

VARIATIONS Other ingredients you can add include chopped green peppers, finely chopped chilli peppers (if tolerated), cheeses (including dairy-free variants), or sautéed chopped mushrooms. A good tip is to fry a teaspoon of the mixture to check the taste and seasoning before you cook the loaf.

Chilli con carne

This is what I would call a family Chilli con carne, rather than a purist's version that bans tomatoes and beans. It's a joyous dish that is gloriously "everything free", as indeed are nearly all of the accompaniments suggested below. Great debates break out about the merits of minced beef versus chopped beef and red peppers versus green, so not wanting to cause ructions, I've put in both as options.

    dairy, egg, gluten & nut free

1 tbsp corn or nut-free
   vegetable oil
2 onions, finely chopped
2 garlic cloves, finely chopped
1 red or green pepper, deseeded
   and diced
2 tsp hot chilli powder or 2 tbsp
   mild chilli seasoning
½ tsp chilli flakes
½ tsp ground cumin
450g (1lb) lean beef, minced or
   cut into small cubes

1 x 400g (14oz) can of chopped
   tomatoes
200ml (7fl oz) tomato purée
200ml (7fl oz) water
1 x 400g (14oz) can of red kidney
   beans, drained and rinsed
salt to season

PREPARATION TIME 12 minutes
COOKING TIME 2 hours
SERVES 4

SERVING SUGGESTIONS Serve with cornbread (pp.174–76) or boiled long grain rice. Top with wedges of fresh lime, parsley, chopped avocados, tomatoes, spring onions, guacamole, and salsa.

Soured cream and grated Cheddar or Monterey Jack cheese are traditional accompaniments. If you are allergic to dairy, use non-dairy soured cream and buy some of the excellent non-dairy Cheddar and Monterey Jack cheeses available.

1 Heat the oil in a flameproof casserole dish. Fry the onion, garlic, pepper, and spices gently for about 4 minutes, until the vegetables are softened and lightly golden.
2 Add the beef and fry until browned. If using mince, use a wooden spoon and turn constantly to break up any lumps.
3 Add the remaining ingredients and season to taste. Bring to the boil, reduce the heat, cover, and simmer gently for 1 hour, stirring occasionally. Remove the lid and continue to simmer until rich and tender, a further 1 hour, stirring occasionally to prevent sticking. Taste and re-season if necessary.

WATCH OUT FOR chilli as some people can't tolerate it. Leaving out chilli and chilli flakes turns it into something closer to a ragu – still good, but definitely not a chilli con carne.

TIPS This is a great do-ahead dish, as it improves with reheating.
   You can make this serve 5–6 people by adding another drained can of red kidney beans.
   The amount of chilli powder is very much a matter of taste. This version is fairly hot. You can use pure chilli powder or the milder chilli seasoning, which is a mix of chilli with other spices and oregano. Add as little or as much as you like.

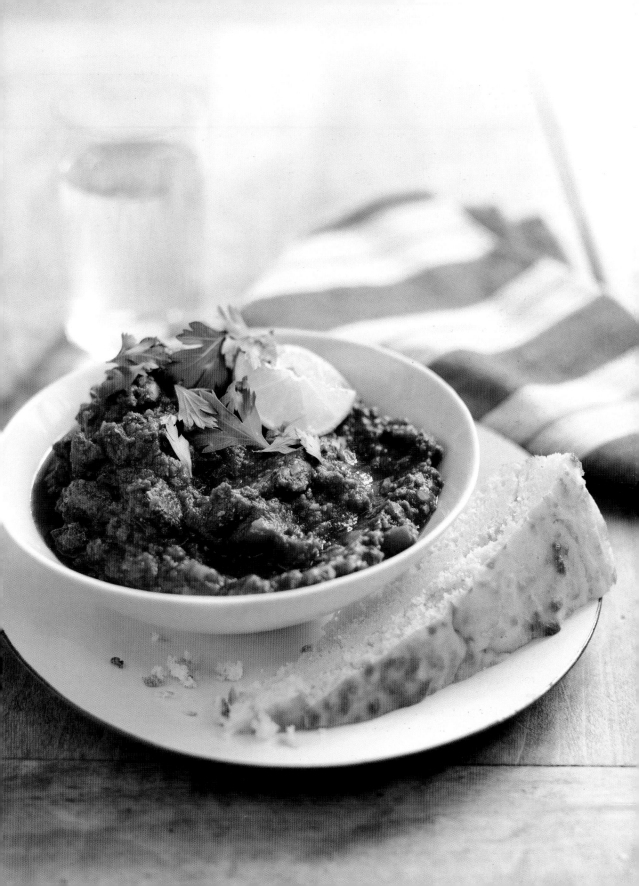

Vietnamese beef stew

This delicious aromatic beef stew is warming enough for a winter supper, yet smart and unusual enough for entertaining. The Vietnamese excel at subtle mixtures that are fragrant rather than spicy. Here, the fresh ginger, lemongrass, curry, and chilli powders blend during cooking into a rich brown sauce. You won't believe the delicious, cinnamon-scented aroma that fills the room when you make this.

    dairy, egg, gluten & nut free

for the marinade
2 tbsp grated fresh ginger
2 lemongrass stalks, trimmed
  and very finely chopped
2 tsp mild curry paste or powder
2 tsp ground cinnamon
2 tsp light brown sugar
4 tbsp tomato purée
2 red chillies, deseeded and
  finely chopped
2 tbsp Thai fish sauce
for the stew
900g (2lb) lean stewing steak,
  cubed
3 tbsp corn or other nut-free oil

1 large onion, chopped
3 garlic cloves, crushed
750ml (1¼ pints) water
1 tsp salt
2–4 star anise
freshly ground black pepper
2 carrots, cut into chunky pieces
2 potatoes, cut into chunky pieces
1 daikon or 2 small turnips, cut into
  chunky pieces

PREPARATION TIME 15 minutes
  plus marinating time
COOKING TIME 1½ hours
SERVES 4–6

1 Mix all the marinade ingredients together in a large bowl. Add the meat and toss with your hands to coat completely. Leave to marinate for at least 1 hour or overnight.

2 Heat 1 tablespoon of the oil in a flameproof casserole dish. Add the onions and garlic and fry, stirring, until softened and translucent, about 2 minutes. Remove from the dish with a draining spoon.

3 Heat the remaining oil in the dish. Add half the meat and brown quickly on all sides. Remove from the dish. Add the remaining meat and brown quickly. Return the rest of the meat, any remaining marinade, and the onions and garlic to the pan.

4 Stir in the water and add the salt and star anise. Add a good grinding of pepper. Bring to the boil, reduce the heat, cover and simmer very gently for 1 hour.

5 Add the prepared vegetables and simmer gently until everything is tender, a further 30 minutes.

6 If necessary, remove the lid and boil the stew rapidly for 1–2 minutes to reduce the liquid slightly. Taste and re-season if necessary. Serve straight from the pot.

TIP As with most stews, this tastes even better when made in advance and then reheated, making it perfect for dinner parties.

SERVING SUGGESTIONS Serve the stew with rice and Asian slaw (p.212). To create a stylish meal with an Eastern flavour that works for all "Big Four" food allergies, serve with Fresh spring rolls (p.90) as a starter, and end with Coconut sorbet (p.159). This stew is also delicious over noodles or scooped up with French bread (pp.170–171).

WATCH OUT FOR chilli as some people can't tolerate it. Omit if need be.

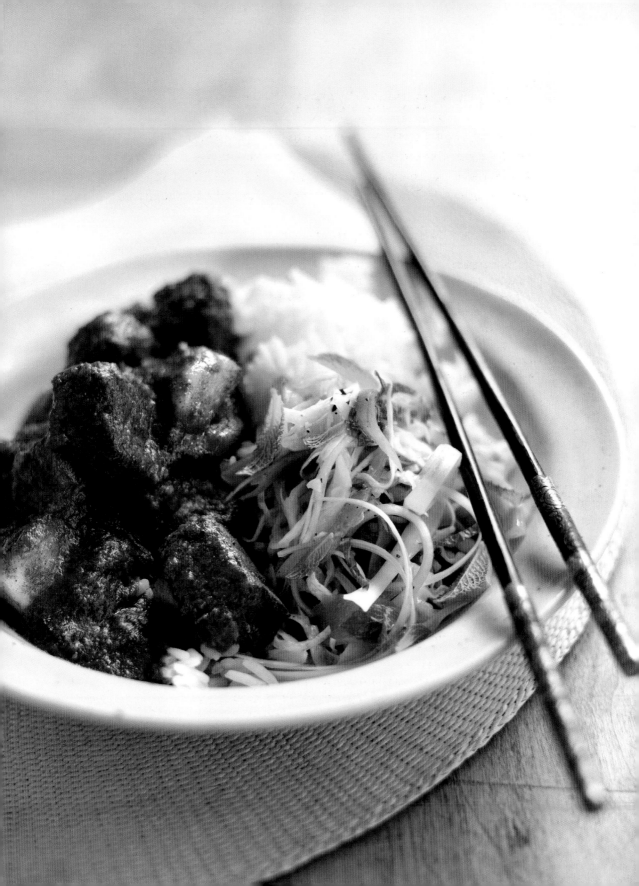

Chinese-style spare ribs

Serve these sticky, delicious glazed ribs on a big plate for everyone to help themselves. Roast in the oven, or part-cook and then barbecue. If you like, serve them on a bed of shredded Chinese leaves (or other lettuce) and top with spring onions and toasted sesame seeds. Kids love these, but they're definitely finger food, so paper napkins and finger bowls are strongly recommended.

   dairy, egg & nut free

for the marinade
4 tbsp soy sauce
2 tbsp rice vinegar
4 pieces of stem ginger
   preserved in syrup, drained
   and very finely chopped or
   crushed in a garlic crusher
4 garlic cloves, crushed
150ml (5fl oz) Hoisin sauce
1 tsp five-spice powder
1.8kg (4lb) pork spare ribs
   (450g/1lb per person), cut
   into separate ribs

to garnish
sliced spring onions
sesame seeds (optional)

PREPARATION TIME 8 minutes plus
   marinating time
COOKING TIME 1½ hours
SERVES 4

1 Mix the marinade ingredients in a large non-metallic or glass shallow dish. Add the ribs and turn to coat. Leave in the fridge to marinate for at least 3 hours, turning the ribs occasionally.
2 Preheat the oven to 190°C (375°F, gas 5).
3 Place a sheet of foil in a roasting tin and transfer the ribs and their marinade to the foil. Wrap loosely.
4 Roast in the oven for 1 hour. After an hour, open up the foil and turn the ribs over.
5 Increase the oven temperature to 220°C (425°F, gas 7) and roast with the foil open for a further 30 minutes or until the ribs are sticky and glazed. Turn the ribs once.
6 Serve immediately.

TIP To barbecue, follow the recipe up to step 5. Roast the ribs for 1 hour and transfer to the barbecue to finish. Brush with the remaining marinade just before barbecuing. You can cook them from raw, but they won't be as tender. Cook slowly on the barbecue (not too near the coals) as too high a heat will caramelize the sugars in the marinade and burn.

 gluten free
also dairy, egg & nut free

Follow the recipe on the left, but make sure that you use a gluten-free soy sauce. Also, some brands of Hoisin sauce may contain malt vinegar or wheat products, making them unsuitable for gluten-sensitives. If that is the case, you can make your own as follows, but note the cautions below.
Hoisin sauce
4 tbsp gluten-free soy sauce
4 tbsp black bean or yellow bean paste
2 tbsp molasses
2 tsp rice vinegar
¼ tsp garlic powder
2 tsp sesame oil
¼ tsp chilli sauce (optional)
a good grinding of black pepper
Mix all of the ingredients together until smooth.

WATCH OUT FOR sesame seeds. If you are allergic to them, omit from the garnish and use corn oil instead of sesame oil if you are making the Hoisin sauce. Some people cannot tolerate chilli, so omit the chilli sauce if necessary. Check that the black bean or yellow bean paste does not contain gluten.

FISH, MEAT & POULTRY

Roast pork with fennel

Fennel and pork are a winning combination. In this dish, they're paired in two ways, with fennel seeds coating the joint and bulb fennel cooking around it. The pan juices make a delicious gravy. Serve the pork with carrots and Roast potatoes with garlic & sea salt (p.95) for a perfect Sunday lunch or supper. This is an easy meal to shop for as the recipe uses a cut of meat that is readily available in supermarkets.

    dairy, egg, gluten, & nut free

3 fennel bulbs
6 tbsp light olive oil
1 tbsp light brown sugar
1.1 kg (2½lb) boned pork loin
  (skin removed, but fat left on)
1 tsp rock salt
1 tbsp crushed black peppercorns
3 tbsp fennel seeds
1 tbsp finely chopped fresh
  rosemary

240ml (8fl oz) vegetable or
  chicken stock
240ml (8fl oz) dry white wine
lemon juice (optional)

PREPARATION TIME 10 minutes
COOKING TIME 1 hour 40 minutes
  (including gravy)
SERVES 6–8

TIPS Pork loin is a lean cut and can overcook and dry out easily so buy meat with a layer of fat on top and leave it on during cooking.

If you like crackling, roast the skin alongside the joint. Score the skin, sprinkle with salt and place on a flat baking tray. Roast on a high shelf for 20–30 minutes or until it is crisp.

WATCH OUT FOR stock cubes, which may contain traces of dairy or gluten, if you're cooking for people with severe dairy or gluten sensitivities.

1 Preheat the oven to 190°C (375°F, gas 5).

2 Cut off the feathery fronds from the fennel. Cut the bulbs lengthways into quarters or sixths, depending on their size.

3 In a bowl, toss the fennel pieces in 4 tablespoons of the olive oil and brown sugar to coat them evenly.

4 Tie the pork with string at regular intervals in four or five places along its length, so that it is cylindrical. This will give you a more evenly cooked and better looking roast.

5 Heat the remaining oil in a roasting tin. Brown the joint quickly all over. Mix together the rock salt, peppercorns, fennel seeds, and rosemary on a large flat plate, spreading it out evenly. Roll the joint in this mixture, pressing it into the joint with your hands.

6 Place the joint on a rack in the roasting tin. Arrange the fennel pieces around the joint.

7 Roast in the oven until cooked through and the fennel is golden and caramelized at the edges, but still slightly firm in the centre, about 1½ hours. Turn the fennel once during cooking.

8 Transfer the pork and fennel to a carving dish and keep warm. Spoon off the excess fat from the roasting tin, leaving the juices. Add the stock and wine and stir, scraping any bits stuck to the pan into the liquid using a wooden spoon. Strain the gravy into a saucepan to remove any stray seeds or peppercorns. Boil rapidly for 5 minutes until reduced by half. Season and sharpen with lemon juice, if liked.

9 Carve the pork, transfer to warm plates, and spoon the gravy over.

Moussaka

This famous Greek speciality is an excellent do-ahead dish, particularly if you have a large number to feed. The layers of aubergines, lightly spiced minced beef, and creamy béchamel sauce should be served bubbling hot and it needs no more than a crisp salad to accompany it. I've suggested feta or Parmesan in the béchamel, but other cheeses, including dairy-free ones, work very well too.

  ### egg & nut free

3 aubergines
salt
olive oil
2 large onions, chopped
3 garlic cloves, finely chopped
½ tsp ground cinnamon
¼ tsp paprika or mild chilli powder
500g (1lb 2oz) minced lamb
1 tbsp tomato purée
200ml (7fl oz) red wine

freshly ground black pepper
½ tsp dried oregano
6 tbsp plain flour
1 quantity Béchamel sauce (p.208)
75g (2½oz) crumbled feta or grated Parmesan

PREPARATION TIME 1¼ hours
COOKING TIME 40 minutes
SERVES 6

1 Cut the aubergines lengthways into 5mm (¼in) slices. Place in a colander, sprinkle with salt, and leave for 30 minutes for the salt to draw out the bitter juices; then rinse and pat dry with kitchen paper.
2 Heat 2 tablespoons of olive oil in a heavy-based casserole dish or frying pan and fry the onions and garlic for 2 minutes until softened. Stir in the spices.
3 Add the minced lamb and fry until browned. Using a wooden spoon, turn the mince constantly to break up any lumps. Add the tomato purée and wine, season with salt and pepper, and stir well. Bring to the boil, reduce the heat as low as possible, and simmer uncovered, stirring occasionally, for 40 minutes. Remove from the heat and stir in the oregano.
4 Meanwhile, heat enough olive oil to coat the base of a frying pan, season the flour with salt and pepper, and dip the aubergine slices in the flour. Fry in batches until golden on each side. Drain well on kitchen paper.
5 Make the béchamel sauce and stir in the feta or Parmesan.
6 Preheat the oven to 190°C (375°F, gas 5). Line the base of a 20 x 25cm (8 x 10in) ovenproof dish with a layer of aubergine slices, then half the meat, then aubergines, then the remaining meat, finishing with aubergines. Top with the béchamel sauce. Bake for 40 minutes until the top is lightly browned and bubbling.
Pictured opposite ▶

 ### dairy free
also egg & nut free

Follow the recipe on the left, but use the dairy-free Béchamel sauce recipe. Use dairy-free crumbled feta or dairy-free grated Parmesan, Gouda or Cheddar-style cheese.

 ### gluten free
also egg & nut free

Follow the recipe on the left, but substitute rice flour for plain flour when coating the aubergine slices and use the gluten-free version of Béchamel sauce.

WATCH OUT FOR chilli, as some people can't tolerate it. Omit the chilli powder if need be.

TIP Do not stint on the kitchen paper when draining the oil from the cooked aubergine, as this prevents the moussaka from swimming in oil.

SERVING SUGGESTION Serve with a mixed salad topped with olives and cubes of feta cheese or a dairy-free alternative.

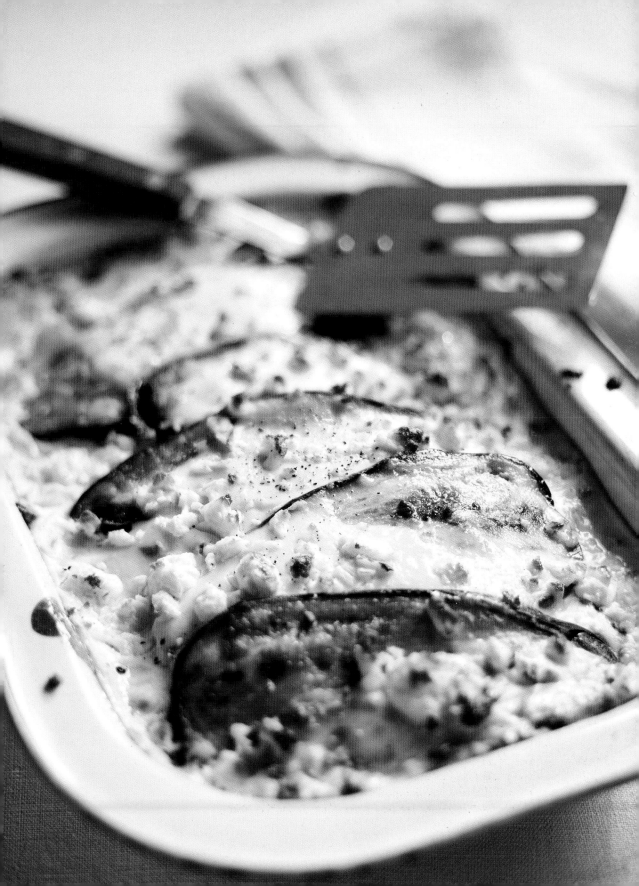

Classic shepherd's pie

A universally popular combination of minced lamb with finely chopped onion, celery, and carrots, simmered under a topping of floury mashed potatoes, with a dusting of nutmeg. Making shepherd's pie has never been an exact science, so add in chopped leftover roast meat and vary the vegetables and seasonings to taste; some people swear by the addition of peas and ketchup to the mince.

  egg & nut free

3 tbsp nut-free vegetable oil
1 onion, chopped
1 celery stick, finely chopped
2 carrots, coarsely grated or finely diced
1 tbsp chopped fresh thyme
750g (1lb 10oz) minced lamb
150ml (5fl oz) beef or vegetable stock
1 tbsp plain flour
1 tsp Worcestershire sauce
1 tbsp tomato purée
1 bay leaf

salt and freshly ground black pepper

for the potato topping
1.25kg (2½lb) floury potatoes, peeled, quartered, and rinsed
55g (2oz) butter
1 tbsp milk
large pinch of freshly grated nutmeg

PREPARATION TIME 50 minutes
COOKING TIME 45 minutes
SERVES 4–6

1 Heat 2 tablespoons of the oil in a heavy-based pan and fry the onion, celery, carrot, and thyme for about 5 minutes, stirring, until softened. Remove from the pan and reserve.
2 Heat the remaining oil and fry the lamb until evenly browned, stirring constantly with a wooden spoon to break up the meat.
3 Add the stock and flour to the meat. Add the reserved vegetable mixture, Worcestershire sauce, tomato purée, bay leaf, and seasoning to taste.
4 Bring to the boil, stirring, until thickened. Reduce the heat, cover, and simmer very gently, stirring occasionally, for 30 minutes, until tender. Transfer to a shallow ovenproof serving dish, discarding the bay leaf.
5 Meanwhile, cook the potatoes in boiling, lightly salted water for about 15 minutes, until tender. Drain and mash with 45g (1½oz) of the butter and the milk using a potato masher or a fork. Season with nutmeg and salt and pepper to taste.
6 Preheat the oven to 180°C (350°F, gas 4). Spread the potatoes over the top of the meat mixture, roughing up the surface with a fork for a crispier topping, and dot with the remaining butter.
7 Bake for about 45 minutes until piping hot and the potatoes are lightly browned.

 dairy free
also egg & nut free

Replace the butter with dairy-free spread and the milk with soya or rice milk or oat milk. Check the stock is dairy free.

 gluten free
also egg & nut free

Follow the recipe on the left, but at step 3 substitute 1½ teaspoons (half the quantity) of cornflour for the ordinary flour and blend until smooth with 1 tablespoon of water. Mix into the meat and stock.

TIP Use leftover cooked meat if preferred and adjust the seasoning.

WATCH OUT FOR stock cubes, which may contain traces of dairy or gluten. Make sure the Worcestershire sauce is gluten free if need be.

FISH, MEAT & POULTRY

Spinach & yogurt lamb curry

This Indian curry is redolent of the heady aromas of the subcontinent. With a base of onions, garlic, cumin, coriander, and cloves, the lamb is simmered slowly in fresh ginger, spinach, and yogurt until it is tender and almost falling apart. Just add rice and raita (p.213) and you have a real feast for the senses. Best made a day ahead and reheated.

   egg, gluten & nut free

120ml (4fl oz) flavourless nut-free oil
2 onions, finely chopped
1½ tsp ground cumin
1 tsp ground coriander
pinch of cayenne
pinch of ground cloves
1 bay leaf
4 garlic cloves, crushed
2.5cm (1in) piece of fresh ginger, grated
675g (1½lb) boned lamb shoulder or neck fillets, cut into 2.5cm (1in) cubes

150ml (5fl oz) plain yogurt
675g (1½lb) fresh or thawed frozen leaf spinach
salt and freshly ground black pepper
¼ tsp garam masala
2 tbsp chopped fresh coriander

PREPARATION TIME 10 minutes
COOKING TIME 45–60 minutes
SERVES 4

 dairy free

also egg, gluten & nut free

Substitute soya yogurt for the dairy yogurt. If serving with raita, use the dairy-free version.

WATCH OUT FOR cayenne pepper, which is chilli based. Some people cannot tolerate chilli, so omit if in any doubt.

1 Heat the oil in a large, heavy-based casserole dish and fry the onions for 2 minutes, stirring until softened but not browned.
2 Add the cumin, coriander, cayenne, cloves, and bay leaf and fry gently for 1 minute, stirring.
3 Add the garlic and ginger and fry for a further minute. Add the meat and fry for 2 minutes, stirring, until browned all over.
4 Add the yogurt and mix well. The yogurt will curdle, but don't worry, it forms a rich sauce at the end.
5 If using fresh spinach, trim, wash, and roughly chop. If using frozen, squeeze out any excess water. Add the spinach to the pan. Stir and cook until the spinach has softened and wilted. Season with salt and pepper.
6 Cover and simmer very gently until the meat is tender, 45–60 minutes. Skim any excess oil from the top. If cooking ahead, allow to cool to room temperature, then chill overnight.
7 To serve, reheat gently, if necessary, stirring until piping hot. Stir in the garam masala and coriander and serve with boiled rice or flatbreads (gluten-free if necessary), chutney, and raita (see p.213).

Honeyed Welsh lamb

We spend a lot of time on our farm in Wales, which supplies organic lamb and beef to supermarkets. This recipe shows off delicious late summer Welsh lamb and honey – and is really a tribute to locally produced food. The cider gives a subtle apple taste to the gravy and the glaze roasts to a rich brown. Serve with leek-flavoured, Gratin gallois (p.94) and seasonal vegetables.

    dairy, egg, gluten & nut free

1 tbsp flavourless nut-free oil
4 tbsp clear honey
4 tsp finely chopped fresh
   rosemary
1 tsp grated fresh ginger
1.8–2kg (4–4½lb) leg of lamb,
   preferably Welsh!
4 tbsp dry cider
for the gravy
juices from the meat
150ml (5fl oz) meat or
   vegetable stock

½ tsp cornflour (optional)
salt and pepper to season

PREPARATION TIME 10 minutes
COOKING TIME 2–2½ hours
SERVES 6–8

TIP You need plenty of foil to prevent the honey glaze dripping into the roasting tin, where it's likely to burn and impart a bitter taste to the gravy.

WATCH OUT FOR stock cubes, as they may contain traces of dairy or gluten.

1 Preheat the oven to 190°C (375°F, gas 5).
2 In a small bowl, mix together the oil, honey, rosemary, and ginger to form a thick paste.
3 Using a skewer, stab holes in several places on the surface of the lamb. Rub the honey mixture over the meat.
4 Cut a piece of extra-wide foil – big enough to wrap the leg of lamb loosely. Place the foil in a large roasting tin and place the leg of lamb on top. Pour the cider around the base of the lamb. Loosely fold the foil around the joint and secure the edges.
5 Roast for 2–2½ hours, basting twice with the juices during the cooking. This timing will give you pink lamb.
6 Remove the roasting tin from the oven, put the lamb onto a plate and leave to relax in a warm place for 20 minutes. Keep the meat juices in the tin and discard the foil.
7 To make the gravy, place the roasting tin on a moderately hot stove, add the stock to the meat juices and simmer until thickened. If a thicker gravy is preferred, spoon a little of the hot stock into a cup and then stir in ½ teaspoon of cornflour until smooth. Return the mixture to the roasting tin and stir until thickened. Season with salt and pepper to taste. Keep warm until ready to serve.

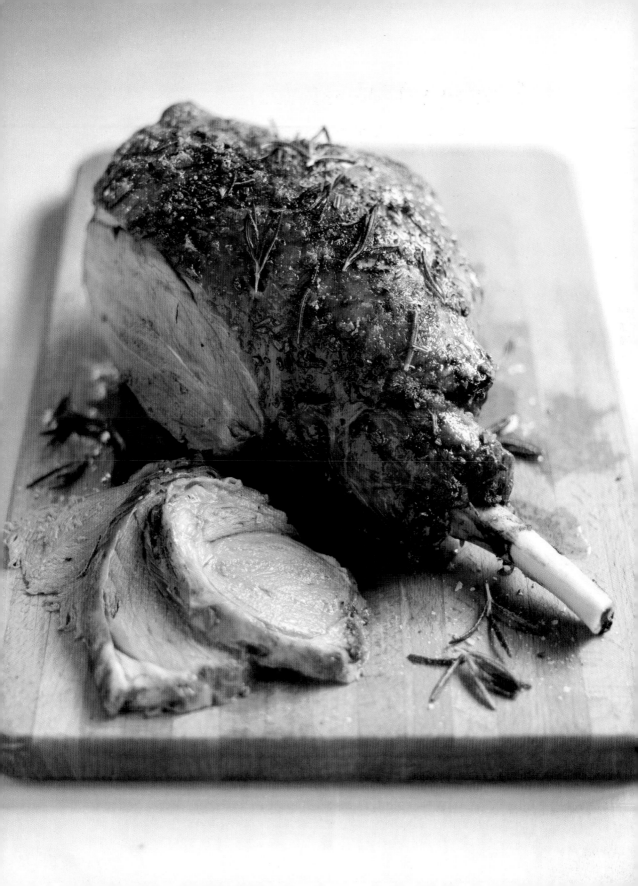

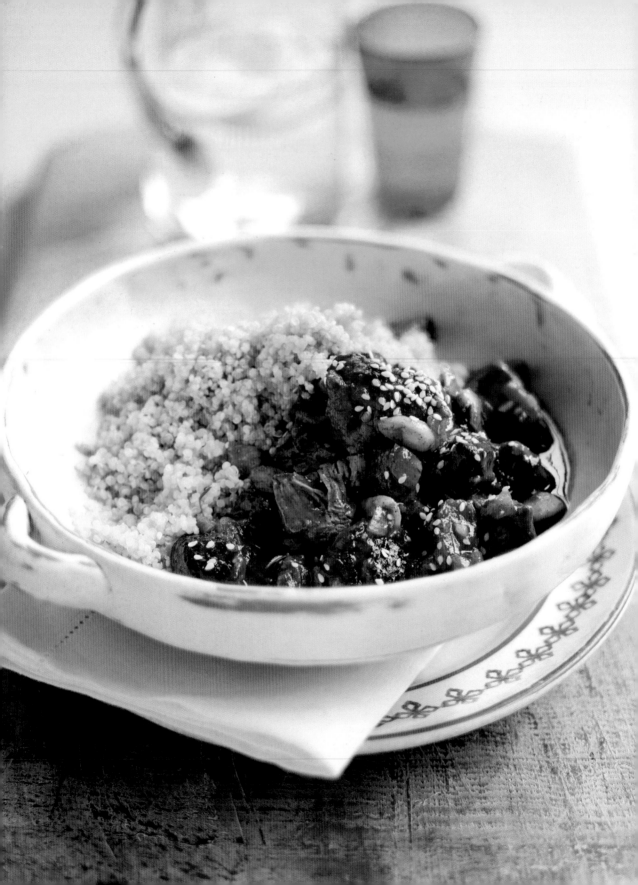

Lamb tagine

A savoury-sweet combination of fruit, nuts, and meat gives this fragrant stew the characteristic taste of Morocco. It's best to use stewing cuts such as neck or shoulder, and to simmer it as long and low as possible. Couscous is the traditional accompaniment, but the saffron quinoa couscous is a terrific alternative – whether you need to be gluten free or not.

  dairy & egg free

4 tbsp light olive oil

900g (2lb) stewing lamb, ideally from the shoulder or neck, cut into 2.5cm (1in) cubes

1 onion, finely chopped

2 garlic cloves, finely chopped

1 tsp ground cumin

1 tsp ground cinnamon

½ tsp ground ginger

500ml (17fl oz) vegetable or meat stock

1 tbsp clear honey

2 tbsp tomato purée

5cm (2in) piece of orange peel

1 cinnamon stick

salt and pepper to season

85g (3oz) pitted prunes, halved

85g (3oz) dried apricots, halved

55g (2oz) blanched almonds, lightly toasted

1 tsp orange flower water (optional)

to garnish
sesame seeds

for the couscous
225g (8oz) couscous

300ml (10fl oz) boiling water

PREPARATION TIME 20 minutes

COOKING TIME 1¼–1½ hours

SERVES 4–6

1 In a large heavy-based, flameproof casserole dish, sear the lamb pieces, a few at a time, in 2 tablespoons of the oil. Remove the browned pieces with a draining spoon and set aside.

2 In the same pan, on a medium-low heat, fry the onions and garlic in the remaining oil until softened but not browned (about 2 minutes). Stir in the ground spices and cook for a minute longer.

3 Return the lamb to the casserole dish, and add the stock, honey, tomato purée, orange peel, and cinnamon stick. Mix well and season with salt and pepper. Bring to the boil and then reduce the heat. Simmer, part-covered, for 1–1¼ hours. Stir in the prunes, apricots, almonds, and orange flower water, if using, and cook, covered, for a further 15 minutes or until the dried fruit has absorbed some liquid and has softened.

4 Meanwhile, put the couscous in a bowl, add a pinch of salt, and pour the boiling water over. Stir well. Place the bowl over a pan of gently simmering water. Cover and leave until the water has been absorbed, at least 5 minutes, or until the tagine is ready.

5 Fluff up the couscous with a fork, spoon onto warm plates, and serve with the tagine. Garnish with sesame seeds.

 nut free

also dairy & egg free

Follow the recipe on the left, but replace the almonds with an equal quantity of toasted pine nuts, if these are tolerated. If in any doubt, do not use.

 gluten free

also dairy & egg free

Follow the recipe on the left, but make saffron quinoa couscous as follows:

• Heat 800ml (1⅓ pints) of lightly salted water. Add ¼ teaspoon of powdered saffron or ½ teaspoon of saffron threads and stir.

• Bring to the boil, add 300g (10½oz) quinoa, and reduce to a simmer. Cook, covered, for about 10 minutes (the quinoa is cooked when the germ separates and you can see a tiny thread-like white tail on each grain). Remove from the heat and leave to stand for 10 minutes.

• Fluff up with a fork before serving.

◄ Pictured opposite

WATCH OUT FOR stock cubes. Check that they are dairy free or gluten free as necessary. Some people are allergic to sesame seeds, in which case omit.

Lasagne al forno

A classic dish of pasta sheets layered with a rich meaty ragu and béchamel sauce and dusted with Parmesan. The ragu and béchamel can be made in advance and the dish assembled on the day. If you can't find gluten-free pasta sheets, use the recipe on the next page. Or do as the Italians do and layer thin slices of pre-cooked polenta in place of the pasta to create a *polenta pasticciata*.

  ## egg & nut free

for the filling
1 quantity Ragu Bolognese (p.117), omitting the chicken livers and cream and increasing the minced beef to 400g (14oz)

for the topping
1 quantity Béchamel sauce (p.208)
55g (2oz) Parmesan, grated

to finish
280g (10oz) precooked egg-free lasagne sheets

PREPARATION TIME 2½ hours (including cooking the Bolognese)
COOKING TIME 35–40 minutes
SERVES 4–6

1 Make the ragu Bolognese according to the instructions on page 117 and above.
2 Make the béchamel sauce according to the recipe on page 208.
3 Preheat the oven to 190°C (375°F, gas 5). Put a spoonful of the meat mixture in the base of a 1.4 litre (2½ pint) ovenproof dish and spread it out. Top with 2 lasagne sheets. Layer half the meat, then two more sheets of lasagne, then the rest of the meat and top with the last two sheets of lasagne. Spoon the béchamel sauce over and sprinkle with the Parmesan.
4 Bake in the oven until bubbling and turning golden on top, 35–40 minutes. Serve hot.

SERVING SUGGESTION A fresh green or mixed salad is the perfect accompaniment to lasagne.

 ## dairy free
also egg & nut free

Follow the recipe on the left, but use 1 quantity of the dairy-free version of Béchamel sauce (p.208). Top with 55g (2oz) of grated dairy-free Parmesan equivalent.
Pictured opposite ▶

 ## gluten free
see recipe overleaf

If you can't find gluten-free pasta sheets in the shops or by mail order, use the simple recipe overleaf. Alternatively, layer thin slices of pre-cooked Polenta (p.81) in place of pasta.

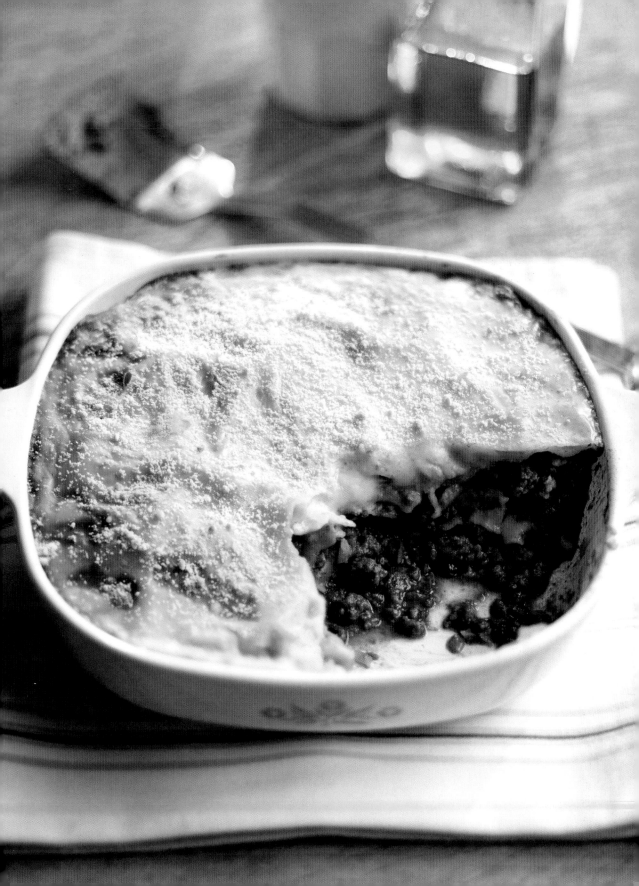

Lasagne al forno continued

 gluten free
also nut free

for the lasagne sheets
85g (3oz) gluten-free plain white
  flour plus extra for dusting
¾tsp xanthan gum
¼tsp salt
1 large egg, beaten
1 tbsp olive oil

PREPARATION TIME 2¾ hours
(including making the pasta and
cooking the Bolognese)
COOKING TIME 35–40 minutes
SERVES 4–6

1 Prepare as for the nut- and egg-free recipe on page 136, but
  make the pasta first. Sift the flour with the gum and salt in a
  bowl. Work in the egg and oil to form a firm dough.
2 Knead gently on a work surface until smooth. Wrap in cling
  film and leave to rest for 30 minutes.
3 Roll out the dough as thinly as possible and cut into six
  15 x 7.5cm (6 x 3in) sheets, re-kneading and rolling the
  trimmings as necessary. Lay the sheets on a board to dry while
  you make the filling. Continue as for the nut- and egg-free
  recipe on the previous page.

TIPS Try using buckwheat flour
instead of gluten-free white flour.
  You can also cut the rolled-out
dough into thin ribbons for home-
made tagliatelle. Leave it to dry for
30 minutes then simply boil it in
lightly salted water for a few
minutes until just tender.

"If you've never
made pasta before,
you'll be surprised
how easy this is"

Haddock & spinach pasta bake

This is a proper old-fashioned supper dish; creamy pasta layered with smoky haddock and spinach, enhanced with spring onions and mushrooms, and the whole lot topped off with tomatoes and cheese. It can be made in advance and then just put in the oven to brown when you're nearly ready to eat. If you're making the gluten-free version, I recommend it with corn pasta.

  ## egg & nut free

250g (8½oz) undyed smoked haddock
300ml (10fl oz) milk
225g (8oz) dried durum wheat, egg-free pasta shapes
30g (1oz) butter
1 bunch of spring onions, finely chopped
55g (2oz) button mushrooms, sliced
30g (1oz) plain flour
4 tbsp single cream

1 tbsp lemon juice
2 tbsp chopped fresh parsley
salt and freshly ground black pepper
225g (8oz) leaf spinach, fresh or frozen and thawed, chopped
45g (1½oz) grated Cheddar cheese
2–3 tomatoes, sliced

PREPARATION TIME 20 minutes
COOKING TIME 35 minutes
SERVES 4

1 In a saucepan, poach the fish in the milk for about 5 minutes or until the fish flakes easily with a fork. Lift the fish out and flake, discarding any skin and bones. Reserve the milk for the sauce.
2 Meanwhile, cook the pasta according to packet directions. Drain.
3 Melt the butter in a saucepan. Add the spring onions and gently fry for 2 minutes, stirring, until softened but not browned.
4 Add the mushrooms and fry until softened, about 1 minute.
5 Remove from the heat and stir in the flour. Blend in the fish milk. Return to the heat and bring to the boil, stirring all the time. Simmer for 2 minutes, stirring.
6 Add the cream, lemon juice, and parsley. Fold in the haddock and the cooked pasta. Stir well and season to taste. Be careful with the salt, as both the fish and the Cheddar are quite salty.
7 Preheat the oven to 190°C (375°F, gas 5). Transfer half the pasta mixture to a 1.2 litre (2 pint) shallow ovenproof dish. If using frozen spinach, squeeze the thawed spinach to remove excess moisture. Layer it over the pasta and top with the remaining pasta.
8 Sprinkle with the cheese and arrange the tomatoes around the edge. Bake in the oven for 35 minutes until it turns lightly golden. Serve hot.

WATCH OUT FOR egg in pasta. Dried pasta commonly contains just durum wheat and water, but check the label to make sure.

 ## dairy free
also egg & nut free

Follow the recipe on the left, but substitute dairy-free margarine for the butter; soya, rice, or oat milk for the cow's milk; and soya cream for the cream. You can add an extra knob of dairy-free margarine to enrich the sauce. Use dairy-free Cheddar-style cheese for the topping. You can also mix 4 tablespoons of breadcrumbs with 1 tablespoon of melted dairy-free margarine and sprinkle over the surface instead (or, in addition to) the cheese substitute.

 ## gluten free
also egg & nut free

Follow the recipe on the left, but substitute rice or corn pasta for the wheat pasta, and cornflour or another gluten-free flour for the plain flour.

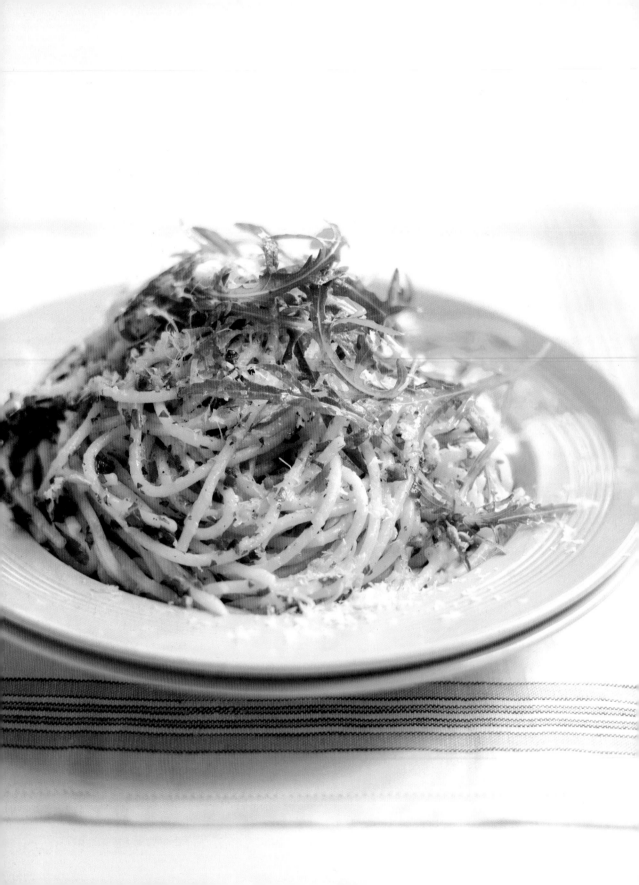

Pasta with rocket

If you like robust modern Mediterranean flavours, this simple-to-prepare but special pasta dish will appeal to you. The piquant garlic, chilli, and lemon mix contrasts well with the peppery rocket leaves and makes for a quick and stylish lunch or supper dish. It can be whipped up in less than 15 minutes: ideal if you have little time to spare for cooking.

  ## egg & nut free

340g (12oz) dried egg-free
   spaghetti
4 tbsp olive oil
4 garlic cloves, finely chopped
1 red chilli, deseeded and
   chopped
zest of 1½ lemons
2 tbsp lemon juice
55g (2oz) rocket torn into 2.5cm
   (1in) pieces or shredded
   finely
30g (1oz) Parmesan, grated plus
   extra to serve
sea salt and freshly ground black
   pepper to season

PREPARATION TIME 3 minutes
COOKING TIME 10 minutes
SERVES 4

1 Cook the pasta in a large pan of boiling water according to the packet instructions or until al dente.
2 Whilst the pasta is cooking, heat the oil in a small pan over a low heat. Add the garlic, chilli, and lemon zest. Cook until the garlic has softened (about 2 minutes). Add the lemon juice.
3 Drain the pasta and pour over the flavoured oil. Add the rocket leaves and parmesan and toss well.
4 Season to taste with salt and pepper and serve immediately, with extra Parmesan on the side.

WATCH OUT FOR chillies, as some people can't tolerate them. Omit if this is the case.

 ## dairy free
also egg & nut free

Follow the recipe on the left, but replace the Parmesan with an equal quantity of non-dairy Parmesan (see Resources, pp.218–219). This can be quite salty so you may need to adjust the seasoning accordingly.
◀ Pictured opposite

TIP If non-dairy Parmesan is not available, try other non-dairy cheeses. An equal quantity of feta-style cheese chopped into 1cm (½in) cubes or non-dairy mozzarella both work well – especially if topped with black olives.

gluten free
also egg & nut free

Follow the recipe on the left, but replace the spaghetti with an equal quantity of a gluten-free version. Corn pasta is ideal in this recipe as it holds the flavours well; 100 per cent buckwheat pasta is fine, too.

Noodles in hot ginger broth

One of the most versatile dishes around, this is a version of the freshly made, comforting, hot noodle bowls served in street stalls and restaurants around the world. Any noodles will work, from Chinese style egg-noodles, to rice noodles or 100 per cent buckwheat noodles for gluten-avoiders. The dish itself cooks in only a few minutes – the ultimate in fast food.

  dairy & nut free

1 litre (1¾ pints) well-flavoured chicken stock
10g (scant ½oz) peeled fresh ginger, cut into fine (julienne) strips
3 tbsp light soy sauce
1 star anise
200g (7oz) noodles
3 tbsp nut-free vegetable oil for stir-frying
8 baby corn, halved lengthways
10 shiitake mushrooms, sliced
2 pak choi, roughly chopped

to garnish
4 spring onions, sliced diagonally
30g (1oz) bean sprouts

PREPARATION TIME 10 minutes
COOKING TIME 12 minutes
SERVES 4

1 Simmer the stock, ginger strips, soy sauce, and star anise for 3 minutes.
2 Cook the noodles according to the pack instructions – until just tender. Divide the noodles between four bowls.
3 Heat a wok until nearly smoking and add the vegetable oil. Stir fry the baby corn to give it a bit of colour and then add the mushrooms and fry for 1–2 minutes.
4 Carefully pour the stock into the wok. Add the pak choi, bring to the boil and simmer for about 1 minute, or until the pak choi is just tender.
5 Ladle the stock and vegetables over the noodles. Garnish with the spring onion slices and a sprinkling of bean sprouts and serve immediately.

 egg free
also dairy & nut free

Follow the recipe on the left, but avoid Chinese or other egg-noodles and use rice noodles, wheat-based udon noodles, or soba buckwheat noodles instead.

 gluten free
also dairy & nut free

Follow the recipe on the left, making sure you use rice, corn, or 100 per cent buckwheat noodles. Make sure the soy sauce is gluten free.
Pictured opposite with wide flat rice noodles ▶

SERVING SUGGESTION Top the noodles and vegetables with 150g (5½oz) of meat, fish, chicken, or duck that has been cut into fine strips and quickly grilled or wok-fried. If you have time, marinate first with sweet miso marinade (see steps 1 and 2 of the recipe on page 101).

WATCH OUT FOR stock cubes, as they may contain traces of dairy or gluten.

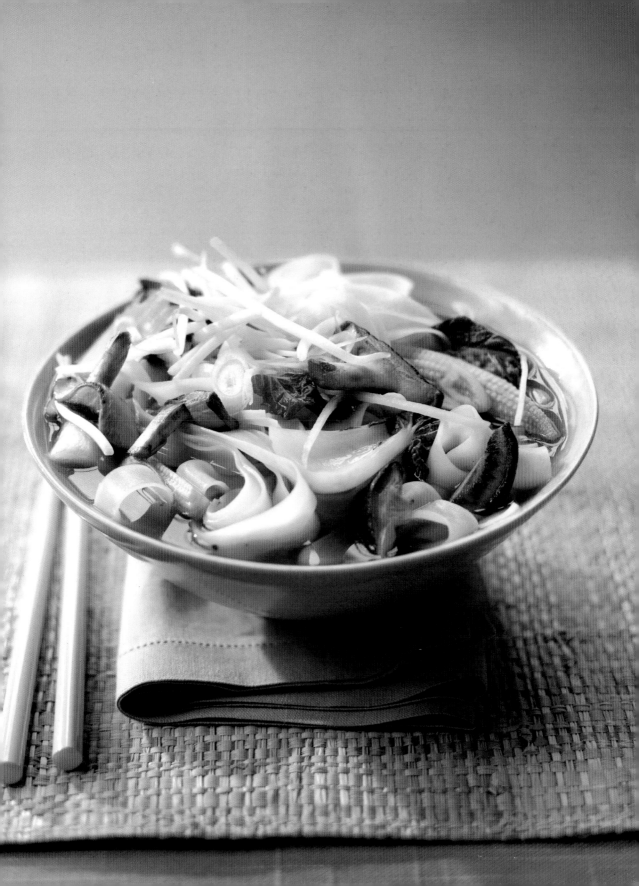

Basmati & wild rice pilaf

This pilaf, studded with dried cranberries, currants and pine nuts is often described as "jewelled" rice, with the basmati and wild rice giving additional contrast to the texture and taste. If you have time, cook the basmati and wild rice separately; if you haven't, buy a mix of wild rice and basmati and start at step two, using all the stock.

    dairy, egg, gluten & nut free

1 litre (1¾ pints) chicken or
   vegetable stock
115g (4oz) wild rice
2 tbsp flavourless nut-free oil
1 onion, finely chopped
1 celery heart, finely chopped
225g (8oz) white basmati rice,
   washed and drained
leaves from 2 sprigs of fresh
   thyme
1 bay leaf
3 tbsp currants

2 tbsp dried cranberries
2 tbsp chopped fresh parsley
3 tbsp pine nuts, toasted
salt and freshly ground black pepper

PREPARATION TIME 10 minutes
COOKING TIME 50 minutes
SERVES 6

TIP If you prefer, use a good knob of butter or dairy-free spread to cook the onions.

1 Put 300ml (10fl oz) of the stock in a saucepan, bring to a boil, and add the wild rice.

2 Cover and reduce the heat to low and simmer for 45–50 minutes until the rice is just tender and has absorbed the liquid (it will still have a nutty texture). If necessary, remove the lid and boil rapidly for a few minutes to evaporate the last of the stock.

3 Meanwhile, heat the oil in a separate saucepan and fry the onion and celery until softened but not browned, 3 minutes.

4 Add the basmati rice and stir until the grains are evenly coated and glistening. Stir in the thyme leaves. Add the remaining stock and bring to the boil. Reduce the heat to low, add the bay leaf, currants and cranberries, and cover and simmer very gently until the rice is tender and the water has been absorbed (about 10–12 minutes).

5 Remove from the heat. When the wild rice is cooked, add to the basmati with the parsley and pine nuts. Season to taste and fluff with a fork.

6 Tip into a warmed serving dish and serve immediately.

WATCH OUT FOR pine nuts, also known as pine kernels, which may not be tolerated by some people who are allergic to nuts. Omit if necessary. If using a stock cube, make sure that it is dairy free and/or gluten free as necessary.

Risotto alla Milanese

An authentic Risotto alla Milanese is a yellow-hued and saffron-scented creamy delight. Serve as a starter or with Osso bucco (p.118). You will need to use short-grain risotto rice and it does take a great deal of stirring, so don't leave it unattended. Use the recipe, minus the saffron, as the basis for your own vegetable, herb, meat, fish or seafood risottos.

   egg, gluten & nut free

1 litre (1¾ pints) chicken stock
150ml (5fl oz) dry white wine
30g (1oz) butter
2 tbsp olive oil
1 onion, finely chopped
30g (1oz) prosciutto ham,
  finely chopped
340g (12oz) risotto rice such as
  arborio or carnaroli
½ heaped tsp chopped saffron
  strands or ½ level tsp
  powdered saffron dissolved in
  2 tbsp hot water
freshly ground black pepper
2 tbsp freshly grated Parmesan
  cheese
salt to taste

PREPARATION TIME 10 minutes
COOKING TIME 20 minutes
SERVES 4

 dairy free
also egg, gluten & nut free

Follow the recipe on the left, but replace the butter with an equal quantity of dairy-free spread, and the Parmesan with an equal quantity of dairy-free Parmesan or other grated dairy-free cheese. For extra creaminess, stir in 2 tablespoons of soya cream alternative in step 3, when adding the saffron.

WATCH OUT FOR stock cubes, as they may contain traces of dairy or gluten.

1 Place the stock and wine in a saucepan and bring to a simmer.
2 In a heavy-bottomed saucepan melt the butter and olive oil and fry the onion and prosciutto until the onion has softened.
3 Add the rice and cook for 2 minutes, stirring well to ensure that each grain is coated with the oil and butter.
4 Add a ladleful of stock to the rice and stir. When the rice has absorbed the stock, add another ladleful. Stir constantly to prevent the rice from sticking. When you have used up half the stock, add the saffron and continue to add the stock, stirring, until all the stock has been used and absorbed, and the rice is tender and creamy, but still firm and with some "bite" to it.
5 Season with freshly ground black pepper. Add the Parmesan and check the seasoning before serving, only adding salt if needed.
Pictured with Osso bucco on page 118

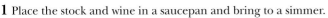

PASTA, NOODLES & RICE

Plum crumble

This is worth making just for the heavenly wafts of autumn fruit, cinnamon, and allspice that fill the kitchen as it cooks. Serve the crumble when the fruit has just begun to bubble through and the topping is barely tinged with brown. Pouring cream, Chantilly topping, custard, or vanilla ice cream are the ideal accompaniments. If nuts are not a problem, try chilled Cashew cream (p.216).

  egg & nut free

for the crumble topping
225g (8oz) plain flour
115g (4oz) cold butter cut into
　2.5cm (1in) pieces
75g (2½oz) soft light or dark
　brown sugar
for the filling
900g (2lb) pitted plums, halved
140g (5oz) granulated sugar
1 tsp ground cinnamon
large pinch of ground allspice

PREPARATION TIME 10 minutes
COOKING TIME 45 minutes
SERVES 4–6

1 Preheat the oven to 190°C (375°F, gas 5).
2 Place the flour in a large bowl. Using the tips of your fingers, rub in the butter until the mixture resembles breadcrumbs. Stir in the sugar.
3 Place the fruit, sugar, and spices in the ovenproof dish and mix to combine. Spoon the crumble mixture on top. Bake for about 45 minutes or until the crumble is golden brown and the fruit is just beginning to bubble through the topping.
Pictured opposite ▶

TIP To ring the changes, try 900g (2lb) of sliced cooking apples, sweetened with 115g (4oz) of sugar plus 2 tablespoons of water, or 900g (2lb) of rhubarb plus 1 tablespoon of chopped stem ginger.

SERVING SUGGESTION Serve with vanilla ice cream, custard, or with dairy-free Chantilly topping or Cashew cream (p.216).

 dairy free
also egg & nut free

Follow the recipe on the left, but replace the butter with an equal quantity of dairy-free spread.

 gluten free
also egg free

Follow the recipe on the left using the following ingredients for the crumble topping:
170g (6oz) gluten-free plain white
　flour mix
85g (3oz) ground almonds
85g (3oz) cold butter, cut into
　2.5cm (1in) pieces
85g (3oz) soft light or dark brown sugar

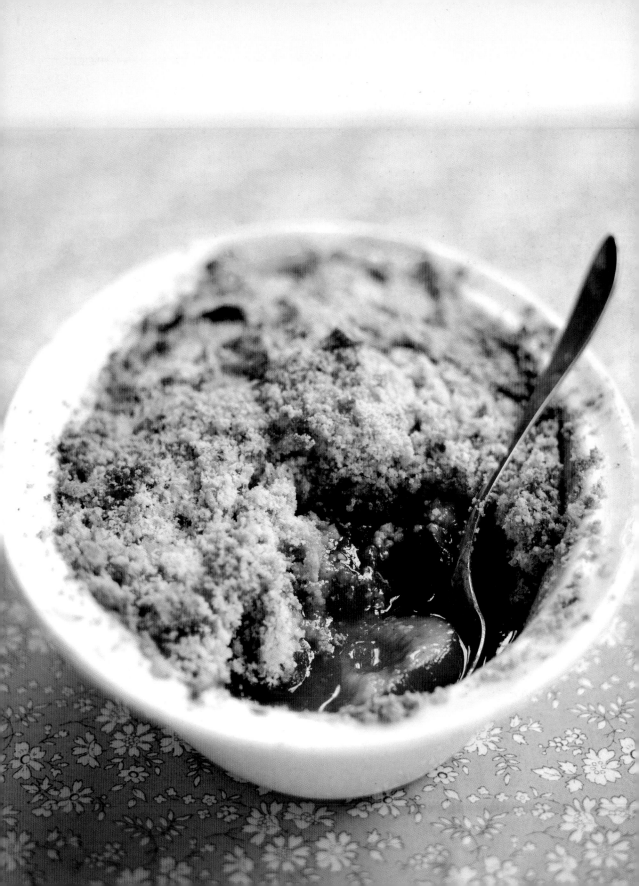

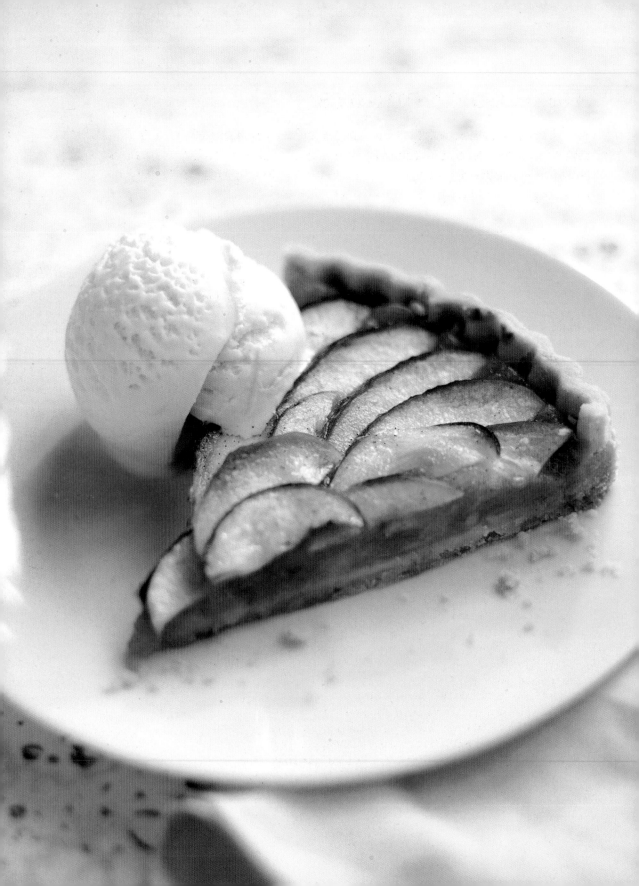

Tarte aux pommes

This delicious classic and versatile Normandy tarte aux pommes works equally well as an elegant dessert or as a stylish tea-time treat. Served warm or at room temperature, the hint of vanilla in the apple is wonderful. Use sharp apples, such as Bramleys or Cox's for the purée and add pretty pink apples for a decorative top layer. Serve with cream or ice cream.

  egg & nut free

1 quantity egg- and nut-free
sweet Shortcrust pastry (p.180),
chilled for 30 minutes
675g (1½lb) eating or cooking
apples, peeled, quartered,
cored, and chopped
200g (7oz) vanilla sugar
1 vanilla pod, split lengthways
450g (1lb) cooking apples
peeled, quartered, cored, and
thinly sliced (about 3mm/⅛in
thick), or rosy eating apples,
thinly sliced with the skin left on

PREPARATION TIME 50 minutes
plus chilling and cooling time
COOKING TIME 1 hour 5 minutes
SERVES 6–8

1 Preheat the oven to 200°C (400°F, gas 6).
2 Roll out the shortcrust pastry and line a 25cm (10in) loose
bottomed tart tin. Place the chopped apples and 55g (2oz) of
the vanilla sugar in a heavy-based saucepan. Scrape the seeds
out of the vanilla pod and add both the pod and the seeds to
the apple and sugar mixture. Cook gently, stirring occasionally,
until the apples are soft and can be pulped when pressed with
a wooden spoon, about 15 minutes. If using eating apples, add
1–2 tablespoons of water to ensure the apples break down easily.
Remove the vanilla pod.
3 Beat the cooked apple well with a wooden spoon, adding
a further 55g (2oz) of the sugar. Leave to cool. Once cool,
transfer to the shortcrust pastry case.
4 Arrange the apple slices in circles overlapping each other on
top of the apple sauce, starting from the outside in.
5 Bake in the centre of the oven for 15 minutes. Remove the tart
from the oven and sprinkle with the remaining 85g (3oz) of
vanilla sugar. Return to a high shelf in the oven and bake until
lightly browned and the sliced apples are tender, about
50 minutes.

 dairy free
also egg free

Follow the recipe on the left, but
use dairy-free sweet shortcrust
pastry (p.180) and serve with soya
cream alternative or dairy-free
ice cream.

 gluten free
also egg & nut free

Follow the recipe on the left, but
use gluten-free sweet Shortcrust
pastry (p.182).
◀ Pictured opposite

TIP If cooking in advance, make the
shortcrust pastry base and freeze it
in its loose-bottomed pan.

SERVING SUGGESTION Serve hot,
warm, or cold, either on its own or
with pouring cream, crème fraîche,
or vanilla ice cream (or a dairy-
free alternative).

DESSERTS

Classic rice pudding

This nursery favourite has enjoyed a surge of renewed popularity recently in restaurants and home cooking. The dairy-free version is a particular delight, as rice milk enhances the flavour further. Using the risotto method (cooking the rice in the butter before adding the milk) gives an even richer and creamier pudding. Flecked with tiny vanilla seeds, this pudding is classy enough to serve at any occasion.

   ## egg, gluten & nut free

15g (½oz) butter
75g (2½oz) granulated sugar
100g (3½oz) pudding or short-grain rice
1 litre (1¾ pints) milk
1 vanilla pod
pinch of salt
150ml (5fl oz) double cream

PREPARATION TIME 10 minutes
COOKING TIME 1½–2 hours
SERVES 4–6

1 Preheat the oven to 160°C (325°F, gas 3).
2 Melt the butter in a 1.5 litre (2¾ pint) flameproof dish on a low heat. Add the sugar and mix well. Add the rice and stir, coating the rice grains with the butter and sugar mixture.
3 Split and scrape the seeds from the vanilla pod. Add the seeds and pod to the milk and stir. Pour the vanilla milk onto the rice and sugar mixture and stir well, using a wooden spoon to break up any lumps.
4 Stir in the salt and cream and bring slowly almost to the boil. Remove the vanilla pod. Transfer to the oven and bake for 1½–2 hours until thick and creamy and browned on top, stirring after 30 minutes and 1 hour.
5 Serve plain or with any of the serving suggestions (right).

TIP For a lighter rice pudding, reduce the amount of double cream to 90ml (3fl oz).

 ## dairy free
also egg, gluten & nut free

Follow the recipe on the left, but replace the butter with an equal quantity of dairy-free spread and replace 1 litre (1¾ pints) of milk with 500ml (17fl oz) of soya milk and 500ml (17fl oz) of rice milk. Replace the cream with an equal quantity of soya cream. If liked, you can use vanilla-flavoured milk and reduce the vanilla to ½ a pod.

SERVING SUGGESTION Serve with cream or soya cream alternative, raspberry or strawberry jam, fruit compôte (see the cherry compôte recipe on page 161), or fruit sauce.

VARIATION Add 2–3 tablespoons of sultanas in step 4 with the cream and salt. Replace the vanilla pod with either the grated zest of ½ a lemon or a good dusting of freshly grated nutmeg.

DESSERTS

Fragrant poached peaches

This is an excellent and versatile way with fruit. I've used peaches but you can also use an equal weight of any stone fruits: apricots, nectarines, or plums. Pears can also be cooked in this way, but take longer. These are all lovely, served in pretty glasses, drizzled with some of the syrup and finished with Chantilly topping (p.216) or ice cream.

    dairy, egg, gluten & nut free

4 peaches (about 450g/1lb),
  unpeeled
240ml (8fl oz) water
225g (8oz) caster sugar
thinly pared zest of ½ lemon
1 vanilla pod

PREPARATION TIME 15–20 minutes
COOKING TIME 5–10 minutes
SERVES 4

1 Cut round the peaches to halve and give a sharp twist to loosen both sides. Lift out the pit or scoop it out with a small knife.
2 Put the water, sugar, and lemon zest in a large, heavy-based saucepan. Split the vanilla pod and scrape out its seeds and add the pod and seeds to the pan. Stir over a low heat until the sugar has dissolved. Bring to the boil and boil for 1 minute. Reduce the heat until the syrup is simmering gently.
3 Add the fruit carefully to the pan. Cover and poach gently for 5–10 minutes, until the fruit is tender when pierced with a cocktail stick or the point of a sharp knife, gently turning the fruit over in the juice halfway through cooking if it is not fully submerged. The poaching time will depend on the ripeness of the fruit. Remove carefully from the pan with a draining spoon, set aside, and keep warm.
4 Boil the juice rapidly for 2–3 minutes, until reduced and syrupy. Remove the vanilla pod. Spoon the juice over the fruit and serve warm.

TIPS For a lighter syrup, reduce the quantity of sugar to 115g (4oz).
  If peeled peaches are preferred, immerse them in boiling water for 10 seconds, then cool immediately in a bowl of cold water. Use a small sharp knife to ease away the skin and brush with lemon juice to prevent discolouration.

VARIATIONS Apricots work well with the vanilla-lemon zest combination (left) and also with brown sugar and a large pinch of white pepper.
  Try poaching plums with a piece of cinnamon stick and the finely grated zest of an orange for a fragrant ruby-red syrup. Star anise and honey also work well with stronger-flavoured fruit.
  Use a little fresh ginger, saffron threads, wine, or spirits to create your own syrup flavours.

SERVING SUGGESTION If there are any leftovers, these desserts are good for breakfast, chopped into granola, blended into smoothies, or grilled briefly under a high heat and served on cinnamon toast.

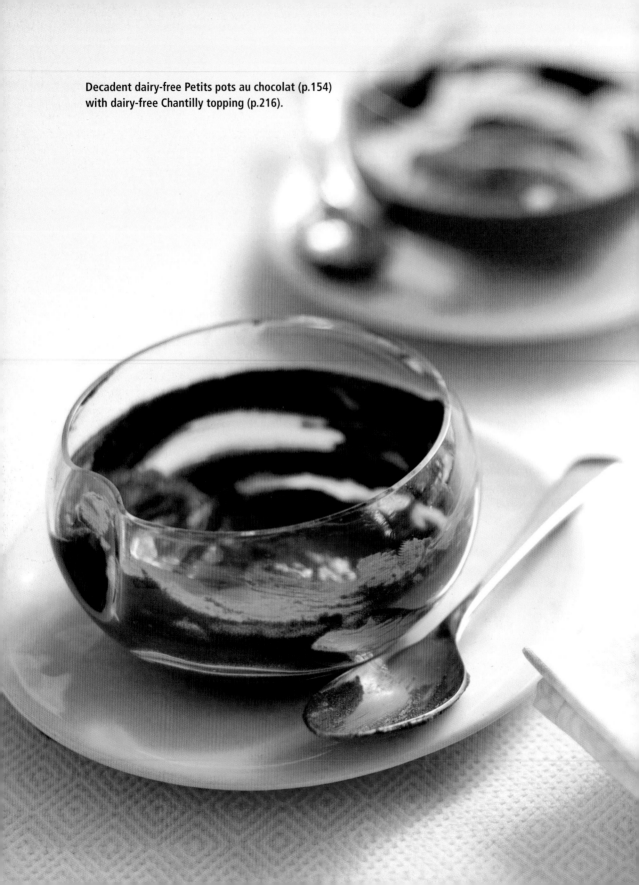

Decadent dairy-free Petits pots au chocolat (p.154)
with dairy-free Chantilly topping (p.216).

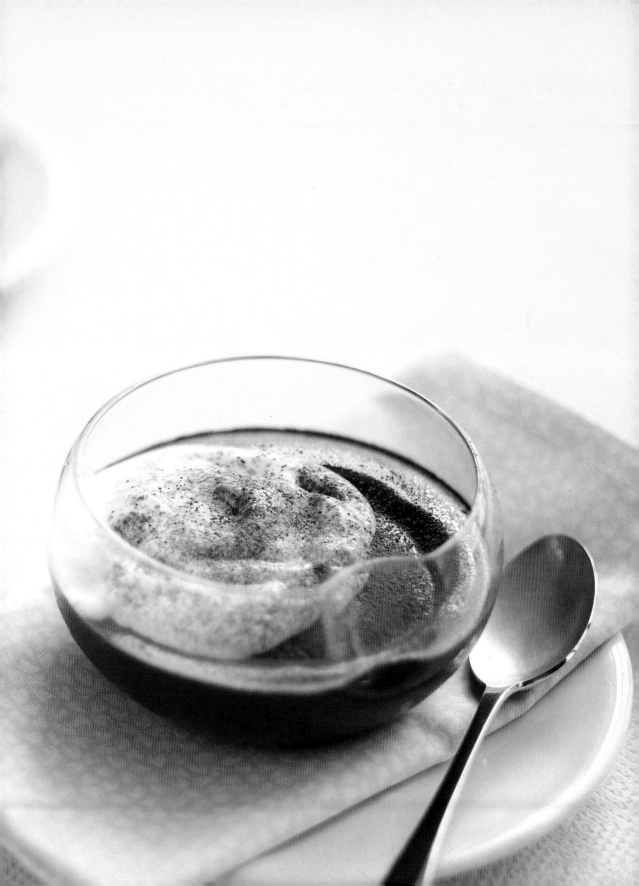

Petits pots au chocolat

These rich, smooth, velvety – very decadent – creations turn eating chocolate into an art form. They're dense and truffley and very simple to make. I serve them in glass dishes but you could also use little demi-tasse coffee cups or small ramekin dishes instead. They are the perfect dessert to linger over and taste as luscious and stylish as they look.

   egg, gluten & nut free

170g (6oz) nut-free plain chocolate with at least 70 per cent cocoa solids
1 tbsp brandy
200ml (7fl oz) double cream
to decorate
4–8 tbsp whipped cream or Chantilly topping (p.216)
1 tbsp nut-free cocoa powder for dusting

PREPARATION TIME 10 minutes plus chilling time
COOKING TIME 10 minutes
SERVES 4

1 Break up the chocolate and place in a bowl over a pan of hot water, ensuring that the bowl does not touch the water. Stir until melted.
2 Warm the brandy and cream in a saucepan until hot but not boiling. Stir into the melted chocolate until completely blended.
3 Spoon the mixture into 4 small ramekins, glass dishes, or demi-tasse cups. Chill until firm.
4 Decorate each with 1–2 tablespoons of whipped cream or Chantilly topping (p.216) and sift the cocoa powder over the top.

SERVING SUGGESTION If you're serving these in demi-tasse cups, decorate each with a chocolate-orange stick, or the little chocolate spoons, which are sold to stir your coffee with.

 dairy free
also egg, gluten & nut free

Follow the recipe on the left, but increase the chocolate to 225g (8oz) (and make sure it is dairy free). Use 150ml (5fl oz) of soya cream alternative instead of the 200ml (7fl oz) of double cream. Decorate with dairy-free Chantilly topping (p.216). ◀ Pictured on previous page with dairy-free Chantilly topping.

Sweet chestnut terrine

This sumptuous, rich dessert is a smart dinner party option because it's so easy to make in advance. Serve it in thin, elegant slices in a pool of luscious, vanilla-flecked cream. Many people who are allergic to nuts are able to tolerate chestnuts so if you know you can eat them, go ahead. If you can't, or are not sure, use the variation at the bottom of the recipe.

   egg, gluten & nut free

a little flavourless nut-free oil
200g (7oz) nut-free plain
  chocolate
185g (6½oz) butter
225g (8oz) caster sugar
1 tbsp brandy
750g (1lb 10oz) cooked peeled
  chestnuts or canned chestnuts
  (drained weight)
120ml (4fl oz) milk

for the vanilla cream

225ml (8fl oz) double cream
2 tbsp icing sugar
½ tsp vanilla extract
½ vanilla pod

PREPARATION TIME 20 minutes
SERVES 8–10

1 Line a 1.2 litre (2 pint) terrine dish or loaf tin with cling film (trying to keep it wrinkle free) or use greaseproof paper and grease with a little oil.

2 Melt the chocolate in a bowl over simmering water, ensuring that the bowl does not touch the water. Add the butter, sugar, and brandy then beat until well mixed. Remove from the heat.

3 In a food processor, purée the chestnuts and the milk to a well-mixed dryish paste.

4 Add the chestnut mixture to the chocolate mixture and mix well until smooth. Pour into the mould, cover, and chill overnight until firm.

5 For the vanilla cream, gently whisk together the double cream, icing sugar, and vanilla extract. Split the vanilla pod and scrape its seeds into the mixture. Do not over-whisk the cream – this is meant to be a pouring cream.

6 To serve, unmould the terrine and use a sharp knife that has been dipped briefly in boiling water to cut thin slices. Pour a small pool of vanilla cream around each portion.

VARIATION If chestnuts are a problem, replace them with an equal quantity of cake crumbs in a cake version that is safe for you.

 dairy free
  also egg, gluten & nut free

Follow the recipe on the left, but substitute equal quantities of dairy-free spread for the butter; and soya milk for the milk in the terrine. Ensure that the chocolate is dairy free. For the vanilla cream, use an equal quantity of soya cream alternative for the double cream, and increase the vanilla extract to 1 teaspoon to mask the strong flavour of the soya cream.

"Rich, dense, and luxurious – an unusual treat for chocolate lovers"

DESSERTS

Green tea ice cream

A deliciously distinctive dessert, Green tea ice cream is often served in Japanese restaurants and is increasingly popular elsewhere. This recipe uses maccha, the finely ground leaves used in Japanese tea ceremonies, or you can make a paler version with green tea leaves. Served on its own or with a drizzle of chocolate sauce, it's a stylish way to round off a meal.

  ## gluten & nut free

2 tbsp maccha green tea powder
300ml (10fl oz) milk
1 vanilla pod
2 egg yolks
100g (3½oz) caster sugar
250ml (8½fl oz) double or
   whipping cream
¼ tsp salt

PREPARATION TIME 20 minutes
COOKING TIME 10 minutes plus
   freezing time
MAKES about 750ml (1¼ pints)

1 Place the maccha green tea powder in a heatproof bowl. Heat the milk to just below boiling point and pour onto the green tea.
2 Stir the mixture to break up any lumps and strain back into the saucepan. Leave to infuse for 15 minutes.
3 Split the vanilla pod lengthways and add to the pan. Heat gently, stirring the vanilla pod to release the seeds. Remove the vanilla pod, scrape out any remaining seeds and add them to the milk, then wash and dry the pod and reserve for future use.
4 Place the egg yolks and the sugar in a medium-sized bowl, and beat with an electric or hand whisk until the mixture is thick and pale. Bring the infused milk back to boiling point and pour it in a thin stream onto the egg yolk and sugar mixture, whisking all the time. Return the mixture to the saucepan and place on the lowest possible heat, stirring continuously as the custard thickens. Cook for 8–10 minutes, stirring, until the custard coats the back of a spoon. Do not allow to boil. The custard will be dark green at this stage.
5 Remove the custard from the heat and leave to cool.
6 Lightly whip the cream with the salt until just softly peaking, but not at all stiff. Fold into the cooled custard with a metal spoon.
7 Freeze in an ice-cream maker following the manufacturer's instructions or pour into a freezerproof container and freeze until just firm around the edges (about 4 hours). Whisk with a fork to break up the ice crystals and freeze until firm. Remove from the freezer 5–10 minutes before serving if hand-made, 20 minutes before serving if made in an ice-cream maker.
Pictured opposite ▶

 ## dairy free
also gluten & nut free

Follow the recipe on the left, but substitute soya, rice, or oat milk for cow's milk and silken tofu or soya cream alternative (which you can whip lightly) for double or whipping cream.

 ## egg free
also gluten & nut free

Follow steps 1–3 of the recipe on the left. You will need just half the quantity of caster sugar used in the other recipes, 50g (1¾oz). Add it to the milk and stir until dissolved. Cool then chill the infused milk and whisk in 5 tablespoons of sweetened condensed milk. Proceed from step 6. This ice cream melts more quickly than the egg-based versions.

TIPS If you can't find green tea powder, infuse 4 green tea teabags in 4 tablespoons of boiling water for 15 minutes. Add both to the hot milk and infuse with the vanilla pod. Squeeze the bags to extract the maximum flavour and colour then discard them. Continue as above or left.

   A quick way to make green tea ice cream is to mix 2 tablespoons of green tea powder with 1 litre (1¾ pints) bought vanilla ice cream.

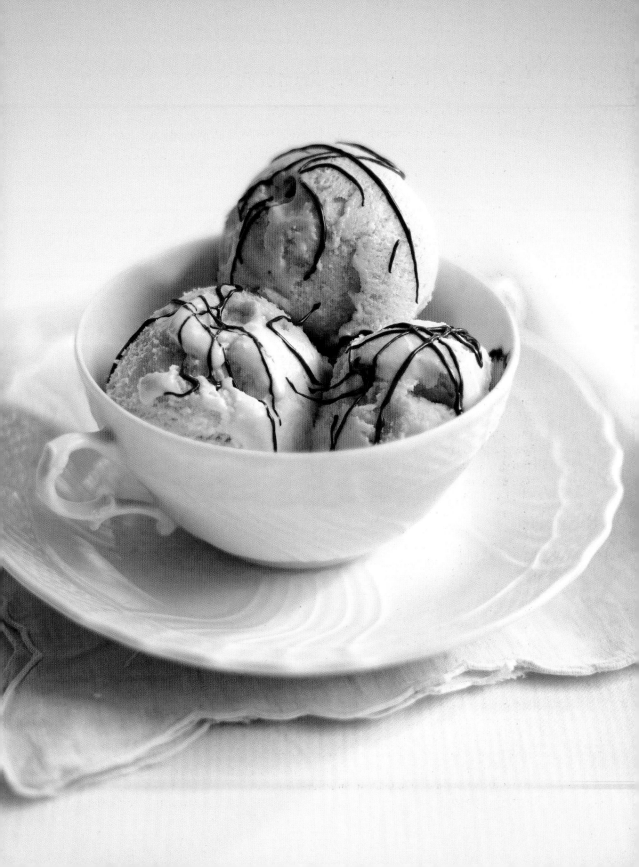

Mango yogurt ice

Mango yogurt ice, flecked with lime zest, is a smooth and intensely fruity dessert. It doesn't take very long to make, and the result is delectably refreshing and incomparably better than the shop-bought variety. The scented tropical fruit makes it the perfect dessert for South East Asian, Indian, or Mexican-inspired food, or for any meal that needs a cool, thirst-quenching finish.

   egg, gluten & nut free

3 ripe mangoes, about
  225g (8oz) each
125g (4½oz) caster sugar
120ml (4fl oz) water
zest and juice of 1 lime
4 tbsp plain yogurt

PREPARATION TIME 5 minutes plus
  chilling and freezing time
COOKING TIME 2 minutes
MAKES about 600ml (1 pint)

1 Extract as much fruit as you can from the mangoes, using a knife to scrape the pulp from the skin and stone. Discard the skin and stone and place the pulp in a measuring jug. You should have around 400ml (14fl oz).
2 In a small saucepan, gently heat the sugar and water and stir until the sugar is dissolved (about 2 minutes). Cool to room temperature. This makes around 200ml (7fl oz) of syrup.
3 In a food processor, blend together the mango pulp, syrup, lime zest and juice, and the yogurt.
4 Place in an ice-cream maker and freeze according to the manufacturer's instructions. Before serving, remove from the freezer and put in the fridge for 20 minutes to soften.

 dairy free
also egg, gluten & nut free

Follow the recipe on the left, but replace the yogurt with an equal quantity of dairy-free yogurt.

TIP If you don't have an ice-cream maker use a freezerproof container, cover and freeze for 3–4 hours or until firm around the edges. Whisk with a fork to break up the ice crystals and freeze again until firm. For a smoother ice cream, repeat the process after an hour or when ice crystals have formed again and then freeze until firm. The Coconut sorbet and Rhubarb sorbet (opposite) can be made in this way too.

"On a hot summer's day this is the nicest thing on earth"

Coconut sorbet

This deliciously creamy sorbet tastes more like a fully-fledged ice cream. Quick and simple to prepare, it is special enough for any occasion and is lovely served with sliced tropical fruits.

    dairy, egg, gluten & nut free

170g (6oz) coconut powder and 600ml (1 pint) water made up into thick coconut milk or
2 x 400ml (14fl oz) cans coconut milk
85g (3oz) caster sugar

1 tbsp desiccated coconut
1 tbsp rum or coconut flavoured rum

PREPARATION TIME 5 minutes plus chilling and freezing time
MAKES about 1 litre (1¾ pints)

TIP It's worth using coconut powder rather than the canned variety if you possibly can as the taste and colour are superior.

WATCH OUT FOR coconut powder. Check the label carefully as some brands contain dairy ingredients.

WATCH OUT FOR coconut allergy. It is very rare, but it is worth asking if you are serving this to people you don't know.

1 In a saucepan, combine the coconut milk with the sugar and desiccated coconut. Over a moderate heat, stir the mixture until the sugar dissolves (about 2 minutes). Add the rum.
2 Allow the mixture to cool to room temperature and chill for at least 30 minutes. Freeze in an ice-cream maker according to the manufacturer's instructions.

Rhubarb sorbet

This sorbet is a lovely delicate dusky-pink colour. Its unexpectedly creamy texture and tangy taste is a triumph and will convert even the most die-hard rhubarb sceptics – children included!

    dairy, egg, gluten & nut free

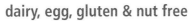

225ml (8fl oz) water
juice of 1 large lemon
140g (5oz) caster sugar
450g (1lb) fresh rhubarb chopped into 2.5cm (1in) pieces
2 tbsp glucose syrup

PREPARATION TIME 15 minutes plus chilling and freezing time
COOKING TIME 8 minutes
MAKES about 1 litre (1¾ pints)

1 Place the water, lemon juice, and caster sugar in a saucepan. Over a low heat, stir until the sugar dissolves.
2 Add the rhubarb, bring to the boil, and simmer for 8 minutes or until the rhubarb is pulpy. Cool to room temperature.
3 Transfer the mixture to a food processor and purée until completely smooth. Stir in the glucose syrup, pulsing briefly for about 25 seconds.
4 Freeze in an ice-cream maker according to the manufacturer's instructions. Remove from the freezer 10 minutes before serving.

DESSERTS

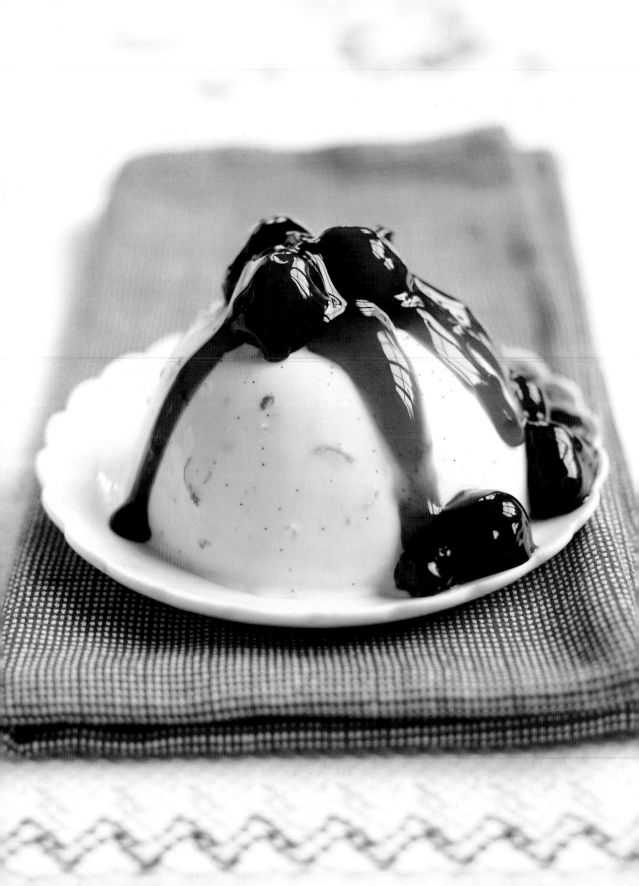

Panna cotta

This dense, creamy Italian speciality is rich and velvety and looks beautiful turned out onto a plate. It gently shimmers, wobbles, and glows in the light and the deep red cherry sauce makes a superlative contrasting accompaniment. It looks good enough for any occasion but don't just keep it for dinner guests, it is an excellent way to round off a light summer lunch, too.

   ## egg, gluten & nut free

nut-free vegetable oil for greasing
2 tbsp hot water
2 tsp powdered gelatine
500ml (17fl oz) double cream
45g (1½oz) caster sugar
1 vanilla pod, split lengthways
thinly pared zest of ½ lime
for the compôte
340g (12oz) fresh cherries, pitted or 1 x 400g (14oz) can of cherries, drained (reserving 3 tbsp of juice)

2 tbsp black cherry conserve
3 tbsp water or juice from canned cherries, if using
2 tbsp icing sugar
juice of ½ lime
3 tbsp brandy
2 tsp cornflour

PREPARATION TIME 30 minutes plus cooling and setting time
SERVES 4

 ## dairy free
also egg, gluten & nut free

Prepare as for the recipe on the left, but use soya cream alternative instead of double cream.

TIP You can also use frozen cherries in this recipe. Thaw them first and prepare in the same way as fresh cherries.

1 Lightly oil 4 individual moulds or ramekin dishes. Put the water in a small bowl and sprinkle the gelatine over. Leave to soften for 5 minutes.

2 Meanwhile, pour half the cream into a saucepan. Add the sugar, vanilla pod, and lime zest and heat gently, stirring, until the sugar has dissolved. Slowly bring almost to the boil and stir in the gelatine until completely dissolved. Remove from the heat and leave to cool.

3 Whip the remaining cream until softly peaked then strain in the cold, flavoured cream; fold in with a metal spoon and transfer to the moulds or ramekins. Chill until set.

4 Meanwhile, make the compôte. Put the cherries in a pan with the conserve, water or juice, icing sugar, and lime juice. Heat gently, stirring until the juices run. If using fresh cherries, cook for 3 minutes only, until the cherries have softened but still hold their shape.

5 Blend the brandy with the cornflour and stir into the cherries. Bring back to the boil, stirring all the time until slightly thickened and clear. Cook for 1 minute then remove from the heat, turn into a bowl, and leave to cool.

6 When ready to serve, gently loosen the edges of the creams with your fingers and then turn them out onto serving plates. Spoon the cherry compôte around and on top of each cream. Serve cold.

◀ **Pictured opposite**

Crêpes

These are the light and lacy French-style pancakes as opposed to the thicker, fluffier American pancakes on page 57. Serve with a squeeze of lemon and sugar, Chantilly topping (p.216), ice cream, and chocolate or toffee sauces, or wrap them around savoury fillings and top with Béchamel sauce (p.208). All versions of the crêpes freeze well – just use greaseproof paper or baking parchment to separate them.

 nut free

115g (4oz) plain flour
¼ tsp salt
2 eggs, lightly beaten
300ml (10fl oz) milk
30g (1oz) butter, melted, plus
  extra for frying

PREPARATION TIME 5 minutes
  plus standing time
COOKING TIME 30 minutes
MAKES 12–15

1 Sift the flour and salt into a large bowl.
2 Make a well in the centre of the flour and whisk in the eggs, gradually drawing in the flour from the sides of the bowl.
3 Pour in the milk, whisk until the batter is smooth and free of lumps. It should now have the consistency of single cream.
4 Stir in the melted butter. Cover and leave the batter to stand in a cool place for at least an hour.
5 Stir the batter again in case any flour has settled at the bottom. Heat the butter for frying in a crêpe pan, or other heavy-bottomed, non-stick frying pan, until hot and tip out any excess, keeping just the barest coating on the pan.
6 Use 1–2 tablespoons of batter for each pancake. Pour in the batter and rotate the pan quickly to ensure the base of the pan is evenly coated with a thin layer.
7 Heat gently for no more than a minute, and when small bubbles appear on the surface use a spatula to flip the pancake.
8 Slide the pancake off the pan onto a plate and keep warm. The pancakes can be stacked and covered with foil to keep warm.

TIPS Make sure you use a non-stick frying pan – this is especially important for the egg-free version. You may need to discard the first pancake or two.

  For sweet pancakes in any version, add 2 tablespoons of caster sugar to the batter in step 3.

 dairy free
also nut free

Follow the recipe on the left, but replace the milk with 300ml (10fl oz) of soya milk. Replace the melted butter with either 2 tablespoons of melted dairy-free spread, or 2 tablespoons of flavourless oil, or 2 tablespoons of coconut cream (coconut milk is too thin). Use a flavourless nut-free oil, such as corn oil, for frying.

 egg free
also nut free

Follow the recipe on the left but replace the eggs with 4 tablespoons of double cream and reduce the quantity of milk to 260ml (9fl oz). **Pictured opposite** ▷

 gluten free
also nut free

Follow the recipe on the left using the following ingredients:
140g (5oz) rice flour
125g (4½oz) tapioca flour
¼ tsp salt
3 eggs, lightly beaten
280ml (9½fl oz) milk
45g (1½oz) butter, melted, plus extra for frying

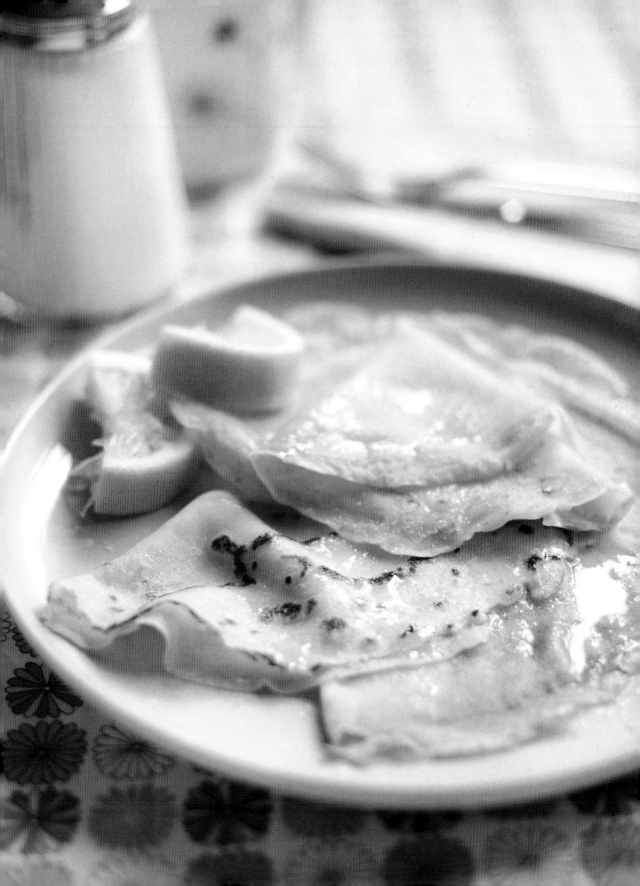

Brown bread

There's been a revival in breadmaking at home. Maybe it's because bread machines make it easier or perhaps it's just the irresistible smell of home-baked bread. Here's a lovely, grainy, seed-studded wholemeal bread. I started making it because there were so many "may contain traces" warnings on manufacturers' and bakery breads, but I now do it for the taste – and the smell!

   dairy, egg & nut free

 gluten free

225g (8oz) strong wholemeal flour
115g (4oz) strong white bread
  flour
55g (2oz) rolled oats
55g (2oz) sesame seeds
30g (1oz) poppy seeds
½ tsp salt
1 tbsp malt extract
2 tbsp olive oil plus a little
  extra for greasing

1 tbsp fast-action dried yeast
280ml (9½fl oz) hand-hot water

PREPARATION TIME 5–10 minutes
  plus rising time
COOKING TIME 30 minutes
MAKES 1 large loaf

The gluten-free version has a super, real bread texture and an excellent flavour. It will even slice thinly for brown bread and butter and sandwiches. See recipe overleaf.

TIP If using a breadmaker, put the wet ingredients in first, then the dry, making sure the malt is nowhere near the yeast (especially if you're putting it on the timer option). Set the machine to "large rapid wholewheat" to cook in the tin, or set it to the "dough" setting. Take out the risen dough from the pan and continue from step 4.

1 Mix the flours with the oats, seeds, and salt in a food processor with a dough attachment or in a bowl.

2 Add the malt, oil, yeast, and water and run the machine until the mixture forms a soft (but not sticky) dough. Run the machine for a further minute to knead the dough. Alternatively, mix the ingredients with a knife and then your hands to form a dough, then turn out onto a lightly floured surface and knead for 5 minutes until smooth and elastic.

3 Place in an oiled polythene bag and leave in a warm place until doubled in bulk (about 45 minutes).

4 Oil a baking sheet or 900g (2lb) loaf tin. Knead the dough again. Either shape into a round and place on the baking sheet or shape into a rectangle and place in the tin. Cover with oiled cling film and leave in a warm place for about 30 minutes, or until well risen.

5 Meanwhile, preheat the oven to 220°C (425°F, gas 7).

6 Remove the film. For the round loaf, score the dough lightly in a criss-cross pattern. Bake in the oven for about 30 minutes until risen, golden, and the base sounds hollow when tapped. Cool on a wire rack.

Pictured opposite ▶

WATCH OUT FOR sesame seeds which some people can't tolerate. If this is the case, use pumpkin seeds in place of sesame seeds, or omit altogether.

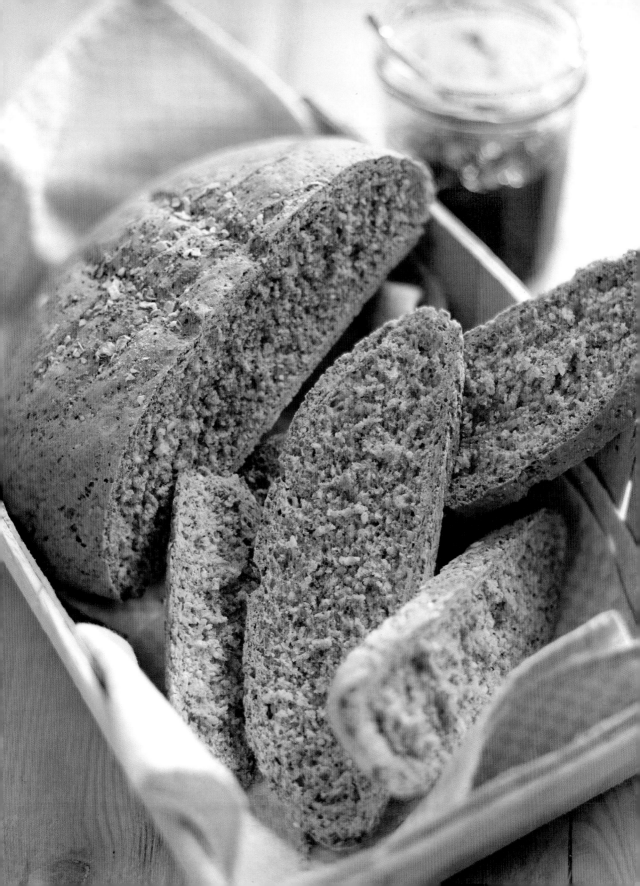

Brown bread continued

 gluten free
also dairy & nut free

300g (10½oz) brown rice flour
20g (¾oz) soya flour
1 tbsp xanthan gum
30g (1oz) sesame seeds
15g (½oz) poppy seeds
1½ tsp salt
1 tsp lemon juice
3 tbsp nut-free flavourless
  vegetable oil, plus a little
  extra for greasing
1½ tbsp molasses
1 tbsp fast-action dried yeast
1 large egg, beaten
400ml (14fl oz) hand-hot water

PREPARATION TIME 6 minutes
  plus rising time
COOKING TIME 40 minutes
MAKES 1 large loaf

1 Oil a 900g (2lb) loaf tin or a deep 20cm (8in) round cake tin.
2 Mix the flours with the xanthan gum, seeds, and salt in a food
  processor (with the ordinary blade attachment) or in a bowl.
  Add the remaining ingredients.
3 Either run the machine until it forms a sticky dough, then run
  it for 1 minute to knead it, or mix everything with a wooden
  spoon or hand beater, beating well for 1 minute once combined.
4 Transfer to the tin and smooth the surface. Cover loosely with
  oiled cling film and leave in a warm place until the dough
  reaches the top of the tin, about 30 minutes.
5 Meanwhile, preheat the oven to 200°C (400°F, gas 6). Remove
  the film and bake in the oven until risen, golden, and the base
  sounds hollow when the loaf is tipped out and tapped, about
  40 minutes. Transfer to a wire rack to cool.

WATCH OUT FOR sesame seeds – some people cannot tolerate them.
If so, simply increase the brown rice flour to 340g (12oz).

TIP You can also make this in the breadmaker. Add the wet ingredients
then the dry. Set the machine to "basic". This isn't suitable for cooking on
the timer.

"This is really quick to make with a healthy, seedy farmhouse texture and taste"

Quick soda bread

Soda bread is the traditional Irish bread and is breadmaking at its quickest; you don't have to wait for yeast to work or the loaf to rise. It makes delicious, crusty, floury bread that can be eaten straight from the oven, broken into farls or quarters, with lashings of butter and jam, and is very popular with coeliac sufferers in the gluten-free form. Soda bread is best eaten on the day it is baked, as it stales quickly.

  ## egg & nut free

225g (8oz) plain flour plus extra for dusting
225g (8oz) wholemeal flour
1 tsp salt
2 tsp bicarbonate of soda
2 tsp cream of tartar
1 tsp caster sugar
45g (1½oz) vegetable shortening or lard

1 x 284ml (9½fl oz) carton of buttermilk
3 tbsp milk, or as needed

PREPARATION TIME 8 minutes
COOKING TIME 50 minutes
MAKES 1 loaf

1 Preheat the oven to 190°C (375°F, gas 5).
2 Sift the flours, salt, bicarbonate of soda, cream of tartar, and sugar into a large bowl. Tip in any bran that remains in the sieve.
3 Using your fingertips, rub the shortening or lard into the flours until the mixture resembles breadcrumbs. Make a well in the centre of the flour mixture and add the buttermilk. Stir with a round-bladed knife, adding enough milk to form a soft, but not sticky dough. You may need more or less liquid depending on the absorbency of the flours you've used. You need to work quickly now, as the raising agents will have started to work once the liquid is added, and you don't want the leavening to finish before you get the dough into the oven.
4 Knead the dough very briefly on a floured surface. Do not spend more than a couple of minutes on this as overworked bread will be tough and heavy.
5 Shape into a 15cm (6in) round, place on a greased baking sheet, and flatten slightly to 5cm (2in) thick. Dust with flour.
6 With a knife dipped in flour, make a deep cross in the top of the bread so that it will break easily into farls when baked.
7 Bake until well risen and brown and the base sounds hollow when tapped, about 50 minutes.
8 Place on a wire rack to cool slightly and cover with a cloth to keep the bread moist.

 ## dairy free
also egg & nut free

Follow the recipe on the left, but use soya yogurt in place of the buttermilk. You can also use soya, oat, or rice milk, replacing 1 tablespoon of the milk with 1 tablespoon of lemon juice or cider vinegar to "sour" it. For either option, have 3 tablespoons of dairy-free milk to hand to help form a soft, but not sticky, dough.

 ## gluten free
also nut free

Follow the recipe on the left, but substitute gluten-free plain white flour for the plain and wholemeal flours, or use half gluten-free plain white flour and half buckwheat flour. Add 2 teaspoons of xanthan gum with the flour and 1 large egg, beaten with the buttermilk.

TIP The buttermilk gives a moist, light loaf and, with the cream of tartar, provides the slightly acid environment that the baking soda needs to work. If you can't get buttermilk, use plain yogurt or the "soured milk" substitution given in the dairy-free recipe above, either with soya milk or dairy milk.

White farmhouse loaf

This is a lovely everyday bread for sandwiches, toast, or cutting into doorsteps to eat with cold meats, pâté, cheese etc. Don't be tempted to cut it before it cools, you'll spoil its lovely soft texture. Making your own bread is worth it just for the taste, but it also means you can avoid the often dubious ingredients, plastic taste, and spongy texture of many factory loaves.

   dairy, egg & nut free

550g (1¼lb) strong white
  bread flour plus extra for
  dusting
2 tsp salt
1 tbsp caster sugar
2 tsp fast-action dried yeast
2 tbsp flavourless nut-free
  vegetable oil plus extra
  for greasing
360ml (12fl oz) hand-hot
  water, or as needed

PREPARATION TIME 5–10 minutes
  plus rising time
COOKING TIME 30 minutes
MAKES 1 large loaf

TIP You can make this in a breadmaker. Put the wet ingredients in first, then the dry, making sure the sugar is nowhere near the yeast – especially if you're using the timer option. Set the machine to the "dough" setting. When risen, take out the dough, transfer to a loaf tin, and continue from step 3.

1 Sift the flour, salt, and sugar into a food processor. Add the yeast and oil and, while running the machine, add enough of the water to form a soft, but not sticky, dough. Run the machine for a further minute to knead it. Alternatively, mix the ingredients in a bowl with a knife, then draw them together with your hands to form a dough. Turn out onto a floured surface and knead until smooth and elastic, 5 minutes.

2 Place in an oiled polythene bag and leave in a warm place until doubled in bulk, about 1 hour.

3 Grease and flour a 900g (2lb) loaf tin. Knock back the dough, re-knead, and shape into a rectangle. Place in the tin, brush with a little water, and dust with a little flour. Cover loosely with oiled cling film and leave in a warm place until the dough reaches the top of the tin, about 30 minutes.

4 Preheat the oven to 230°C (450°F, gas 8). Bake the loaf in the oven for 10 minutes, then reduce the heat to 200°C (400°F, gas 6) and continue to bake until it has risen well above the tin, it is rich brown in colour, and the base sounds hollow when the loaf is tipped out and tapped, about 20 minutes.

5 Cool on a wire rack.

gluten free
also dairy & nut free

400g (14oz) gluten-free plain white flour plus extra for dusting
1 tbsp xanthan gum
1¼ tsp salt
1¼ tbsp demerara sugar
1 tbsp fast-action dried yeast
4 tbsp flavourless nut-free vegetable oil plus extra for greasing
1 tsp lemon juice
1 egg, beaten
400ml (14fl oz) hand-hot water

PREPARATION TIME 5 minutes plus rising time
COOKING TIME 1½ hours
MAKES 1 large loaf

1 Sift the flour, xanthan gum, salt, and sugar into a bowl. Add the yeast, oil, lemon juice, and beaten egg.
2 Add the water and mix to form a thick paste. Beat well with an electric or hand whisk for 2 minutes until smooth. Alternatively, mix in a food processor with the beater attachment for the same amount of time.
3 Transfer the dough to a greased 900g (2lb) loaf tin, dusted with a little gluten-free flour. Smooth the surface. Cover loosely with oiled cling film. Leave in a warm place until the mixture reaches the top of the tin, about 30 minutes. Dust with a little gluten-free flour.
4 Preheat the oven to 200°C (400°F, gas 6).
5 Bake in the oven until risen, richly golden in colour, and the base sounds hollow when turned out and tapped, about 1½ hours.
6 Cool on a wire rack.

TIP For an egg-free and gluten-free version, you can omit the egg and add 2 tablespoons of water, but the texture won't be quite as good.

"This bread is crustier, lighter, and tastier than many shop-bought equivalents"

French-style bread

Commercially produced French bread has a very crisp crust and light texture but does also go stale very quickly. This recipe is not trying to replicate French bakery breads; it has a firmer texture but it slices well, has a good flavour, keeps for several days, and is ideal for freezing. Use it for filled sandwiches, baguettes, canapés, and Crostini (p.72).

   dairy, egg & nut free

a little flavourless nut-free
   vegetable oil for greasing
225g (8oz) strong white flour
³⁄₄ tsp salt
³⁄₄ tsp caster sugar
1 tsp fast-action dried yeast
135ml (4½fl oz) hand-hot
   water, or as needed

PREPARATION TIME 10 minutes
   plus rising time
COOKING TIME 25 minutes
MAKES 1 loaf

1 Oil a baking sheet.
2 Sift the flour with the salt and sugar into a food processor. Add the yeast. Run the machine and add enough water to form a soft but not sticky dough. Continue to run the machine for 1 minute to knead. Alternatively, mix the ingredients in a bowl with a knife, then draw together with your hands to form a dough. Turn out onto a floured surface and knead for 5 minutes until smooth and elastic.
3 Place the dough in an oiled polythene bag and leave in a warm place until doubled in bulk, about 40 minutes.
4 If using a food processor, knock back the dough and re-knead on a lightly floured surface. Shape into a long stick. Place on the baking sheet. Cover loosely with oiled cling film and leave in a warm place to prove again until doubled in bulk, about 25 minutes. Make several slashes along the bread with a sharp knife.
5 Preheat the oven to 200°C (400°F, gas 6). Place a dish of boiling water on the bottom shelf of the oven. Cook the bread on the shelf above the dish until the bread is golden in colour and the base sounds hollow when tapped, about 25 minutes. Brush lightly with water and leave to cool on a wire rack.

SERVING SUGGESTION You can turn this bread into Crostini (p.72) or garlic bread. Cube the last stale little bits and fry them in olive oil for croûtons to sprinkle on soup.

"Using perforated French bread tins makes all the difference to the crust"

gluten free
also dairy & nut free

a little nut-free vegetable oil for
  greasing
150g (5½oz) rice flour
30g (1oz) potato flour plus
  extra for dusting
55g (2oz) tapioca flour
1 tbsp xanthan gum
2 tsp caster sugar
2 tsp salt
1 tbsp fast-action dried yeast
1 egg, separated
1 tsp lemon juice
150ml (5fl oz) hand-hot water, or
  as needed

PREPARATION TIME 8 minutes plus
  rising time
COOKING TIME 40 minutes
MAKES 1 loaf

TIP This gluten-free loaf is not
as light and airy as wheat French-
style bread but slices and toasts
really well. It's best eaten fresh
or sliced and frozen.

1 Mix the flours with the xanthan gum, sugar, and salt into a food
  processor. Stir in the yeast.
2 Whisk the egg white until frothy. Add to the food processor with
  the lemon juice and water.
3 Run the machine to form a soft, slightly sticky dough and
  continue to run the machine for 1 minute to knead the mixture.
4 Turn onto a well-floured surface and knead until no longer
  sticky. Shape into a long stick and place on an oiled baking
  sheet. Cover with oiled cling film and leave in a warm place for
  30 minutes or until doubled in bulk.
5 Meanwhile, preheat the oven to 200°C (400°F, gas 6). Using
  a sharp knife, cut slashes at intervals along the length of the
  bread. Place a dish of boiling water on the lowest shelf of the
  oven. Brush gently with a little of the egg yolk to glaze. Bake
  on the shelf above the dish of water until golden and the base
  sounds hollow when tapped, about 40 minutes. When cooked
  brush lightly with water. Cool on a wire rack.

WATCH OUT FOR rice flours. Some may contain traces of nuts, so
make sure you check the label.

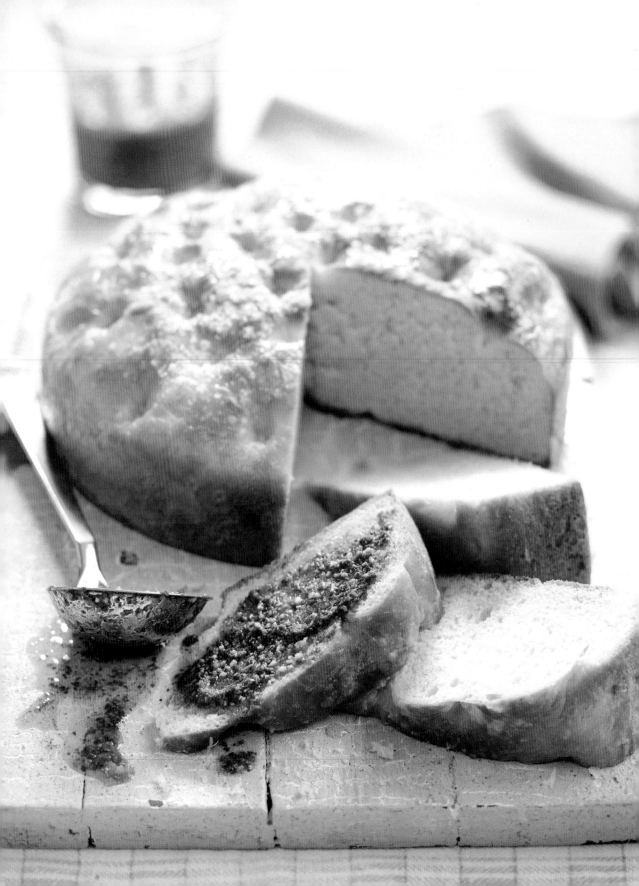

Focaccia

This Italian bread with its soft open texture and dimpled surface is a lovely accompaniment. Serve it plain or try the fragrant seasoned rosemary or basil variations below. It makes a great sandwich bread, too. The main recipe can be baked loaf-like or flatbread-style by varying the proving time; the gluten-free version will not rise quite as high.

dairy, egg & nut free

400g (14oz) strong plain flour plus extra for dusting
2 tsp salt
1½ tbsp caster sugar
1 tbsp fast-action dried yeast
5 tbsp olive oil plus extra for greasing
1 tsp lemon juice

250ml (8½fl oz) hand-hot water, or as needed
1 tsp coarse sea salt

PREPARATION TIME 5–10 minutes plus rising time
COOKING TIME 30 minutes
MAKES 1 round focaccia

1 Sift the flour with the salt and caster sugar into a bowl or food processor.
2 Add the yeast, 3 tablespoons of the oil, the lemon juice, and water. Either mix together with a knife to form a dough then knead on a lightly floured surface for 5 minutes, or run the food processor until a dough is formed and continue to run the machine for 1 minute to knead it to a soft, slightly sticky dough.
3 Lightly oil a 23cm (9in) cake tin and press the dough gently into the tin with wet hands. Lightly sprinkle the dough with water to keep the crust soft. Loosely cover the tin with cling film and leave to prove in a warm place for about 30 minutes or until doubled in bulk. If you like a high loaf, leave it to prove a little longer.
4 Meanwhile, preheat the oven to 220°C (425°F, gas 7).
5 Dust your index finger with flour then gently press it into the dough at intervals to form dimples. Lightly sprinkle with water again, then drizzle with the remaining oil and sprinkle with the coarse sea salt.
6 Bake in the oven until pale golden brown in colour and the base sounds hollow when tipped out and tapped (about 30 minutes). Sprinkle with water twice during cooking.
7 Transfer to a wire rack, cover with a clean damp cloth to soften the crust, and leave to cool.
◄ **Pictured opposite** with dairy-free cheeseless pesto (p.211).

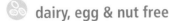 gluten free
also dairy & nut free

Prepare as for the recipe on the left, but substitute gluten-free plain white flour for the strong white flour and add 1 tablespoon of xanthan gum at step 1. Add a beaten egg and increase the water to 330ml (11fl oz). The dough will be sticky. Press it into the tin and smooth the surface with wet hands. Cook for about 45–50 minutes.

VARIATIONS For a rosemary and onion focaccia, follow either recipe, but substitute 1 teaspoon of garlic salt for the plain salt in the dough. Soak 2 thinly sliced onions in cold water for 15 minutes, drain and scatter over the dough and sprinkle with 2 teaspoons of chopped fresh rosemary before drizzling with the oil, sprinkling with coarse sea salt, and baking.

For a sun-dried tomato, olive, and fresh basil focaccia, follow either recipe, but add 2 tablespoons of chopped fresh basil to the dough. When you put the dough back in the tin, chop 4 drained pieces of sun-dried tomato in olive oil and slice 6 pitted black olives. Scatter over the surface of the dough with 6 torn basil leaves, then sprinkle with water and continue at the second half of step 3.

Southern skillet cornbread

Utterly delicious, with a crisp brown crust and golden interior, this cornbread is versatile and quick to make. Eat it on its own, with butter, with Chilli con carne (p.122), flavoured with sweet or savoury additions, served with meals, or in lunchboxes. I've singled out Southern skillet cornbread as it's naturally gluten free, but don't miss out on the four Northern cornbreads overleaf either.

  gluten & nut free

1 tbsp bacon fat or dripping
250g (8½oz) stoneground cornmeal (white cornmeal for preference)
2 tbsp caster sugar
1 tsp baking powder
1 tsp bicarbonate of soda
1 tsp salt
2 eggs, beaten
500ml (17fl oz) buttermilk

PREPARATION TIME 5 minutes
COOKING TIME 20–25 minutes
SERVES 6

1 Preheat the oven to 230°C (450°F, gas 8).
2 Put the bacon fat in a large cast iron skillet or a 23cm (9in) baking tin and heat in the oven.
3 Mix together the cornmeal, sugar, baking powder, bicarbonate of soda, and salt in a large bowl.
4 Whisk together the eggs and buttermilk and add to the cornmeal mixture. Beat until smooth.
5 Pour the batter into the hot bacon fat. Bake towards the top of the oven until the top is browned and the centre springs back when gently pressed, about 20 minutes. Serve immediately cut into wedges.
Pictured opposite ▷

dairy, egg, gluten & nut free

For all four allergen-free versions, there are Northern cornbread recipes overleaf. Sweeter and lighter than its Southern counterpart, Northern cornbread is traditionally baked in a deep tin.

SERVING SUGGESTIONS Eat Southern or Northern cornbreads on their own, with butter, or as an accompaniment to dishes such as meaty stews. Try replacing the sugar with molasses or honey (added to the wet ingredients). Alternatively, add Jalapeño peppers (if you can tolerate them), Monterey Jack, Cheddar or Cheddar-style cheese, or sun-dried tomatoes.

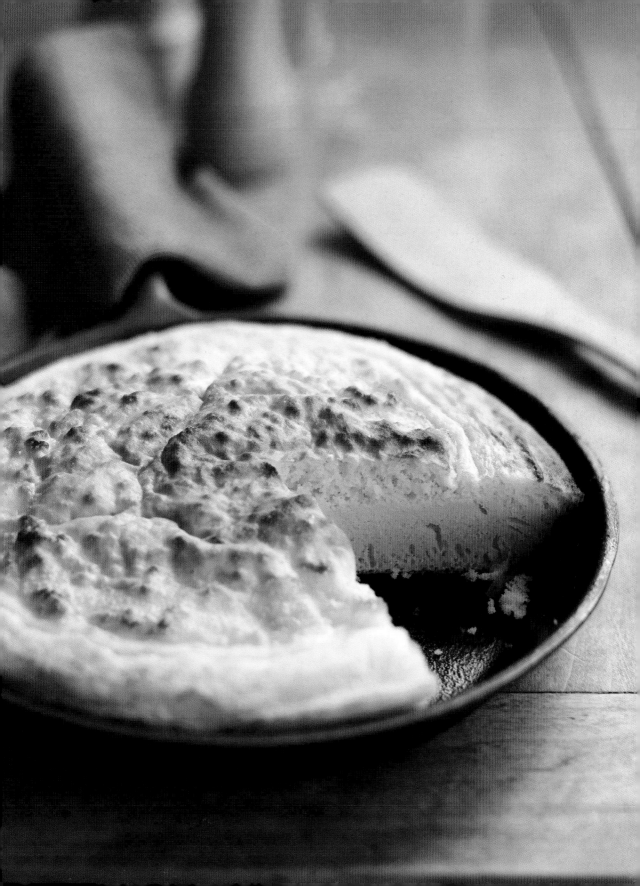

Northern cornbread

 nut free

150g (5½oz) cornmeal
140g (5oz) plain flour
1½ tbsp caster sugar
2 tsp baking powder
½ tsp bicarbonate of soda
½ tsp salt
2 eggs, beaten
140ml (4½fl oz) milk
140ml (4½fl oz) buttermilk
2 tbsp corn oil or 30g (1oz)
  butter, melted

PREPARATION TIME 10 minutes
COOKING TIME 10–12 minutes for
  muffins; 20–25 minutes for tin
SERVES 8–10

1 Preheat the oven to 230°C (450°F, gas 8). Grease a 18 x 23cm (7 x 11in) baking tin or line a standard 12-hole muffin tin with paper cake cases.
2 Mix the cornmeal, flour, sugar, baking powder, bicarbonate of soda, and salt in a large bowl.
3 Whisk the eggs, milk, and buttermilk together and add to the cornmeal mixture. Beat well.
4 Stir in the oil or butter to form a thick paste.
5 Transfer to the prepared tin or paper cases. Bake towards the top of the oven until risen, golden, and firm to the touch – about 10 minutes for the muffins and 20 minutes for the large tin. If baked in the large tin, cut into squares. Serve hot.

TIP For the best flavour, use stoneground yellow cornmeal in this recipe – you can recognize it by the flecks.

 dairy free
also nut free

Replace the milk with an equal quantity of soya milk, and the buttermilk with an equal quantity of soya yogurt. In step 3, stir in corn or vegetable oil instead of melted butter. Proceed as for the nut-free recipe. Remember to grease the baking tin with non-dairy fat or oil. Use dairy-free Monterey Jack or Cheddar-style cheese for variations.

 egg free
also nut free

Omit the eggs. Add 2 tablespoons of soy or potato flour to the dry ingredients and increase the baking powder to 1 tablespoon. Add 3 tablespoons of water and 3 tablespoons of nut-free vegetable oil to the wet ingredients. Proceed as for the nut-free recipe. The egg-free loaf comes out attractively cracked on top and the edges are slightly browner than the nut-free recipe.

 gluten free
also nut free

Prepare as for the nut-free recipe, but substitute gluten-free plain white flour for the white flour and add 1 teaspoon of xanthan gum to the dry ingredients. This doesn't brown as much as the other versions.

Spiced yogurt raisin bread

This spiced loaf is similar to fruited tea breads. Using yogurt instead of milk imparts a nice fresh flavour to the bread. It tastes lovely toasted with butter for breakfast, and try it served with Fragrant poached peaches (p.151). A sliced buttered loaf makes great picnic food too, as it's portable and the flavours are strong enough to hold their own in the fresh air.

  egg & nut free

a little nut-free oil for greasing
340g (12oz) strong white bread flour plus extra for dusting
1 tsp ground mixed spice
½ tsp salt
½ tsp bicarbonate of soda
85g (3oz) soft light brown sugar
1 tbsp fast-action dried yeast
55g (2oz) butter or margarine

280ml (9½fl oz) plain low-fat yogurt
115g (4oz) raisins
a little milk to glaze

PREPARATION TIME 15 minutes plus rising time
COOKING TIME 40 minutes
MAKES 1 large loaf

1 Lightly grease a 900g (2lb) loaf tin and line the base with baking parchment.
2 Sift the flour, mixed spice, salt, and bicarbonate of soda into a food processor or a bowl.
3 Add the sugar and yeast.
4 Melt the butter or margarine in a small saucepan. Stir in the yogurt and heat to warm but not hot. Add to the flour mixture.
5 If using a food processor, run the machine to form a soft, very slightly sticky dough, then run for 1 minute to knead. Turn out onto a lightly floured surface and knead in the raisins. If making by hand, add the raisins to the bowl and thoroughly mix with a wooden spoon, drawing the mixture into a ball. Turn out and knead on a lightly floured surface for 5 minutes until the dough is elastic and no longer sticky.
6 Transfer the mixture to the prepared tin. Cover loosely with oiled cling film and leave in a warm place until the mixture almost reaches the top of the tin, about 1 hour.
7 Meanwhile, preheat the oven to 200°C (400°F, gas 6). Lightly brush the bread with a little milk to glaze and bake in the oven until risen, richly browned, and the base sounds hollow when tipped out and tapped, about 40 minutes. Transfer to a wire rack, remove the baking parchment, and leave to cool.

 dairy free
also egg & nut free

Prepare as for the recipe on the left, but substitute dairy-free spread for the butter or margarine and dairy-free yogurt for the cow's milk yogurt.

 gluten free
also nut free

Prepare as for the recipe on the left, but substitute gluten-free plain white flour for the strong bead flour. Add 1 tablespoon of xanthan gum at step 2 and a beaten egg with the yogurt. The mixture will be quite sticky so, if using a food processor, add the raisins at the end of kneading and just run the machine by pulsating the switch once or twice to incorporate the raisins without chopping them up. You will not be able to knead it on a floured surface so spoon the dough straight into the tin. Leave to rise as in main recipe. Cook until risen, richly browned, and the base sounds hollow when tipped out and tapped. This will take a little longer than the other versions, 50 minutes to 1 hour.

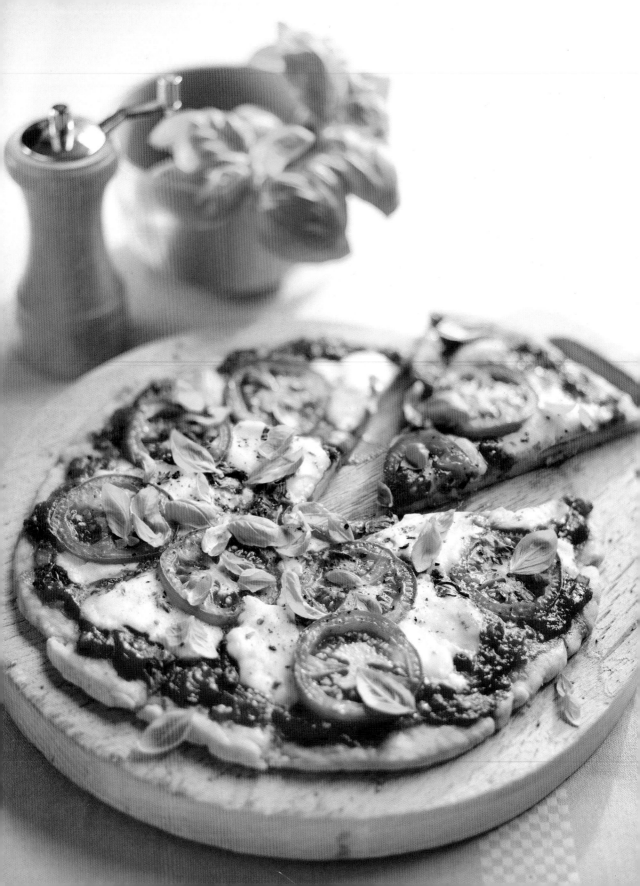

Pizza Margherita

Pizzas are virtually a staple food now and can be tasty, nutritious, and versatile – especially if made at home. This is the classic Margherita with a simple cheese and tomato sauce topping. It's lovely with a handful of wild rocket strewn over just before serving or before baking, add any extra toppings you like, such as anchovies, olives, ham, mushrooms, or roasted vegetables.

 egg & nut free

for the dough
225g (8oz) strong white bread flour
½ tsp salt
1 tsp caster sugar
1 tsp fast-action dried yeast
1 tbsp olive oil plus extra for greasing
120ml (4fl oz) hand-hot water
for the topping
6 tbsp home-made tomato sauce or the best you can buy
1 tsp dried oregano

125g (4½oz) buffalo mozzarella cheese, thinly sliced
3 large tomatoes, sliced
1 tbsp olive oil
freshly ground black pepper
few fresh basil leaves torn into small pieces

PREPARATION TIME 10–15 minutes plus rising time
COOKING TIME 20 minutes
MAKES 1 large pizza

1 Oil a large pizza plate (about 30cm/12in in diameter) or a large baking sheet.
2 Put the flour in a food processor with the salt, sugar, yeast and oil. Run the machine and add the water to form a soft but not sticky dough. Continue to run the machine for 1 minute to knead it. Alternatively, mix the ingredients together in a bowl with a knife to form a dough then turn it out onto a lightly floured surface and knead for about 5 minutes until smooth and elastic.
3 Roll out the dough so that it is about 30cm (12in) in diameter. Transfer to the pizza plate or baking sheet and leave in a warm place to rise for at least 20 minutes.
4 Preheat the oven to 220°C (425°F, gas 7).
5 Spread the tomato sauce over the dough ensuring it doesn't quite reach the edge. Arrange the slices of cheese on top and sprinkle with oregano.
6 Top with the slices of tomato and drizzle with oil and season with pepper.
7 Bake in the oven for about 20 minutes, until crisp and golden around the edges, the cheese has melted, and everything is sizzling.
8 Add a scattering of basil leaves on top.

dairy free
also egg & nut free

Follow the recipe on the left, replacing the buffalo mozzarella with a mozzarella-style melting dairy-free cheese.

 gluten free
also egg & nut free

for the dough
115g (4oz) rice flour
85g (3oz) potato flour
30g (1oz) tapioca flour
1 tbsp xanthan gum
¼ tsp salt
1 tsp caster sugar
1½ tsp fast-action dried yeast
1 tbsp olive oil plus extra for greasing
215ml (7½fl oz) hand-hot water
a little cornflour for dusting
• Oil the pizza plate or baking sheet. Mix the flours with the xanthan gum, salt, sugar, yeast, and oil in a food processor, or mix by hand (see left).
• Add the water and mix to form a soft dough. Continue to run the machine for 1 minute to knead it.
• Transfer to a work surface, dusted lightly with cornflour. Shape the dough into a ball.
• Continue as from step 3 of the main recipe, but cover the dough with oiled cling film to prevent it drying out during rising.
◁ Pictured opposite

Shortcrust pastry

This pastry is the perfect base for fruit tarts such as Tarte aux pommes (p.149) or as a crust for savoury pies like the glazed Chicken pie (p.106). Each version is delicious and has a subtly different texture and hue. If pastry makes you at all nervous, there is advice below as well as specific tips on dairy-free and gluten-free pastry making.

  egg & nut free

250g (8½oz) plain flour plus
   extra for dusting
pinch of salt
140g (5oz) butter, chilled and cut
   into cubes
3 tbsp iced water, or as needed

PREPARATION TIME 10 minutes
   plus chilling time
SERVES 6–8

1 Sift the flour with the salt into a bowl. Using your fingertips, rub in the butter until the mixture resembles fine breadcrumbs.
2 Using a fork or knife, mix with enough cold water to form a soft but not sticky dough. Bring the pastry together completely with your hands.
3 Transfer to a lightly floured surface. Knead gently until smooth and free from cracks. Wrap the pastry tightly in cling film (to prevent the edges from drying out and cracking when the pastry is rolled out) and refrigerate for 30 minutes or until firm. Use as required. It can be frozen.

TIPS The big trick to making shortcrust pastry is to keep everything as chilled as possible – cold room, cold surfaces (a marble board is ideal), cold hands, and cold liquid added to the flour and butter mix.
   You can make your pastry in the food processor, if you prefer. Mix the fat into the flour mixture until just crumbly, but no more. Add the water a little at a time and stop processing as soon as the mixture forms a ball. Do not overmix or the results may be leathery. The less the dough is mixed or handled the better.
   For sweet shortcrust pastry, prepare as above, but add 2 tablespoons of caster sugar with the flour.

 dairy free
also egg & nut free

Follow the recipe on the left, but substitute dairy-free hard white vegetable fat for the butter.

 gluten free

See overleaf for gluten-free recipe.
Pictured opposite ▶

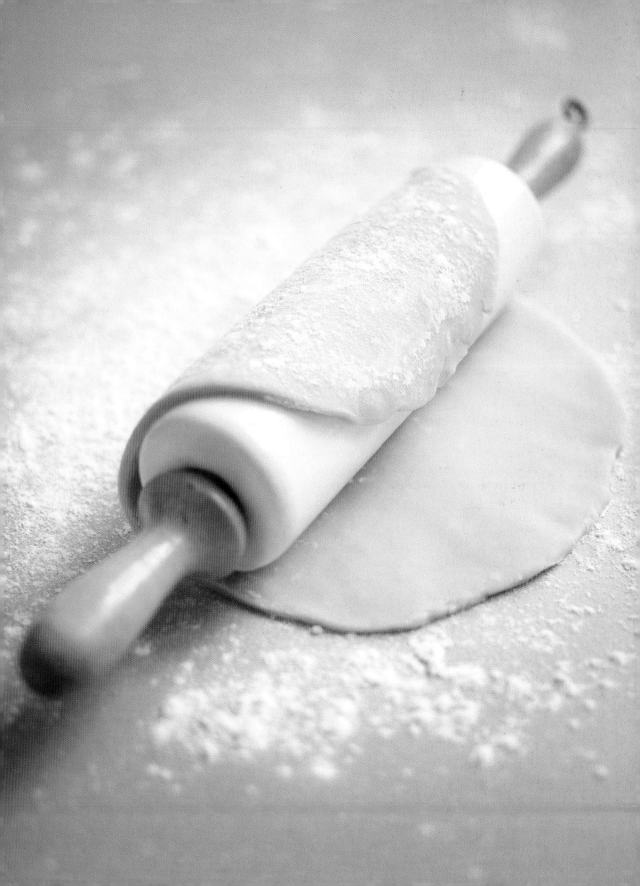

Shortcrust pastry continued

 gluten free
also nut free

115g (4oz) rice flour plus
  extra for dusting
55g (2oz) potato flour
85g (3oz) fine cornmeal
  (polenta)
1 heaped tsp xanthan gum
pinch of salt
140g (5oz) butter, diced
1 egg, beaten with 2 tbsp
  cold water

PREPARATION TIME 10 minutes
  plus chilling time
SERVES 6–8

1 Sift the flours, cornmeal, xanthan gum, and salt into a bowl
  and mix well. Rub in the butter, using your fingertips, until the
  mixture resembles fine breadcrumbs.
2 Make a well in the centre of the mixture and pour about three-
  quarters of the egg and water mixture into it. This should be
  enough to allow you to bring the ingredients loosely together
  with a fork. Add a few more drops if necessary to make the
  pastry come together. Beware of adding more liquid than you
  need; damp pastry may be easier to work with but it may
  toughen up during cooking. Draw the pastry together
  completely with your hands to form a ball.
3 Transfer to the work surface, lightly dusted with rice flour, and
  knead the dough until smooth, about 3 minutes. Shape the
  dough into a ball. Wrap in cling film and chill for 30 minutes
  to rest. Use as required. It can be frozen.

TIPS For sweet gluten-free shortcrust pastry, prepare as above, but add
2 tablespoons of caster sugar at the end of step 1.
  Pastry made with gluten-free flours gives a deliciously satisfying
crumbly crust, but if you are used to regular flours you will find it a little
more difficult to work with. The trick is not to cave in by adding water, but
to work with a dough that has a dryish and crumbly feel to it. That is why
this recipe involves using your hands, as you just don't have the same
degree of control with a food processor.

WATCH OUT FOR rice flour, as it may contain traces of nuts.

Shortbread biscuits

These biscuits are crumbly, delicious, and very moreish. If you find that they don't last long, you might like to make double the quantity. As well as being an ideal snack with a cup of tea or coffee, they work well with fruit desserts. They seem to have a particular affinity to red fruit or berry compôtes and are lovely with strawberries and cream.

  egg & nut free

140g (5oz) softened butter
55g (2oz) caster sugar plus
   extra for dusting
115g (4oz) plain flour
55g (2oz) rice flour
pinch of salt

PREPARATION TIME 25 minutes
   plus chilling time
COOKING TIME 25 minutes
MAKES 10

1 Beat the butter and sugar together until light and fluffy.
2 Sift the flours and salt over the butter and sugar mixture and work in with a wooden spoon until the mixture begins to form a dough.
3 Draw together with your hands to form a soft dough.
4 Knead gently on a board until the mixture forms a ball then roll out with your hands to a sausage about 5cm (2in) in diameter. Wrap in cling film and chill for 1 hour.
5 Preheat the oven to 160°C (325°F, gas 3). Line a baking sheet with baking parchment.
6 Using a sharp knife, cut the sausage into 10 slices and lay them on the baking sheet. If liked, cut with a fluted pastry cutter to give an attractive edge and remove the excess dough. Prick the centres attractively with a fork.
7 Bake in the oven for about 25 minutes until pale golden brown in colour. Remove from the oven and sprinkle immediately with caster sugar. Leave to cool for 10 minutes then transfer to a wire rack to cool completely. Store in an airtight container.

WATCH OUT FOR rice flour, as it may contain traces of nuts.

 dairy free
also egg & nut free

Follow the recipe on the left, but substitute dairy-free spread for the butter and add a few drops of vanilla extract to the mixture to enhance the flavour.

 gluten free
also egg & nut free

Follow the recipe on the left, but substitute gluten-free plain white flour for the ordinary flour.

Raisin scones

Traditionally, scones were part of an elegant tea-time spread served with jam and whipped or clotted cream and quite possibly, Earl Grey tea, too. But you really don't need to get the best linen tablecloth out to enjoy these. They take just half an hour to make, so you can eat them fresh, plain or buttered, with coffee for breakfast, or as a mid-morning snack.

  ## egg & nut free

225g (8oz) self-raising flour plus
  extra for dusting
½ tsp baking powder
¼ tsp salt
30g (1oz) caster sugar
45g (1½oz) butter plus extra
  for greasing
30g (1oz) raisins or sultanas
120ml (4fl oz) milk
2–3 tbsp cream or milk to glaze

PREPARATION TIME 20 minutes
COOKING TIME 10–12 minutes
MAKES 8–10

1 Preheat the oven to 220°C (425°F, gas 7). Grease a baking sheet or line it with baking parchment.
2 Sift together into a medium-sized bowl the dry ingredients: flour, baking powder, and salt. Mix in the sugar.
3 Cut up the butter and rub it into the dry mixture until it resembles fine breadcrumbs. Add the raisins or sultanas.
4 Add three-quarters of the milk and mix it in quickly with a knife. Add the remaining milk, only if it is needed, to mix to a soft dough. Do not overmix as this will make the scones tough.
5 Turn out the dough onto a lightly floured surface and pat or roll out to 2cm (¾in) thick.
6 Cut out the scones with a 5cm (2in) floured cutter. Gather up any trimmings, roll into a ball, and cut more scones.
7 Place the scones on the baking sheet and brush the tops with the cream or milk.
8 Bake near the top of the oven for 10–12 minutes or until the scones have risen, are lightly browned on top, and the bases sound hollow when tapped. Cool on a wire rack.
Pictured opposite ▶

TIP If you like your scones with a soft crust, cover them with a clean tea towel for one minute after removing from the oven.

SERVING SUGGESTION Serve hot or cold with jam and whipped cream or a dairy-free alternative.

 ## dairy free
also egg & nut free

Follow the recipe on the left, but replace the butter with an equal quantity of firm non-dairy spread (the soft ones have too much water in them); and the milk or cream with the same quantity of soya equivalent.

 ## gluten free
also nut free

Follow the recipe on the left, using the following ingredients:
60ml (2fl oz) black tea
30g (1oz) raisins
225g (8oz) gluten-free self-raising flour
½ tsp baking powder
¼ tsp salt
½ tsp xanthan gum
30g (1oz) caster sugar
45g (1½oz) butter
1 egg, lightly beaten
50ml (1¾fl oz) milk
2–3 tbsp cream or milk to glaze

Gluten-free flours can be slightly drier and absorb more water, so make the following alterations. First soak the raisins in the black tea for at least 30 minutes. Add the xanthan gum with the dry ingredients in step 2. Drain the raisins and add to the rubbed-in mixture in step 3. Add the beaten egg before the milk in step 4.

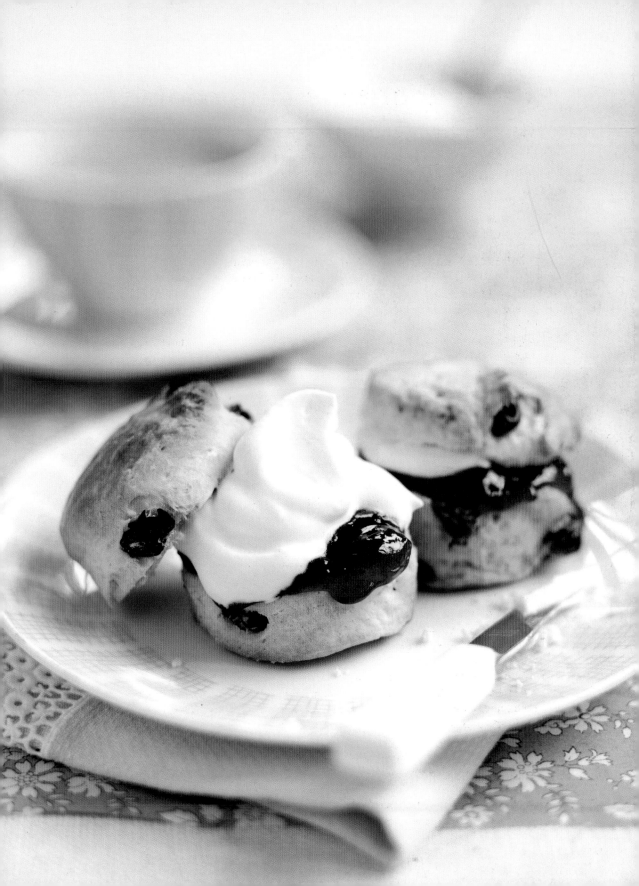

Giant chocolate chip cookies

These thick, golden and chewy cookies, crammed full of chocolate chips, are delicious eaten warm straight from the oven. They seem to be just the right size, giant but not colossal, for children's lunchboxes and look great piled high as part of a tea-time or birthday spread. They also store well and will stay soft if kept in an airtight container.

 nut free

170g (6oz) butter
250g (8½oz) soft light brown sugar
55g (2oz) granulated sugar
300g (10½oz) plain flour
½ tsp bicarbonate of soda
½ tsp salt
1 large egg, beaten
2 tsp vanilla extract
185g (6½oz) bittersweet or semisweet nut-free chocolate chips

PREPARATION TIME 20 minutes
COOKING TIME 20 minutes
MAKES 18 giant or 24 medium cookies

1 Preheat the oven to 180°C (350°F, gas 4). Line two baking sheets with baking parchment.
2 Melt the butter in a small saucepan and add in the sugars, stirring until no lumps remain.
3 Sift the flour, bicarbonate of soda, and salt into a mixing bowl.
4 Add the melted butter and sugars, the beaten egg, and vanilla extract and mix to a soft dough.
5 Mix in the chocolate chips.
6 With wet hands, shape the dough into 18 or 24 balls. Place well apart on the prepared baking sheets.
7 Bake for 20 minutes or until golden and well spread but still slightly soft. Remove from the oven and leave to cool on the baking sheets for 10 minutes then transfer to a wire rack to cool completely. Store in an airtight container.

TIP You can make the dough in advance, roll it into a log and freeze it, ready for cutting into cookies at a later date.

 dairy free
also nut free

Follow the nut-free recipe, but replace the butter with dairy-free spread and add an extra 30g (1oz) of flour. Make sure the chocolate chips are dairy free.

 egg free
also nut free

Follow the nut-free recipe, but omit the egg and replace with 1 tablespoon of potato flour added in step 3 and 3 tablespoons of cream, milk, or water added in step 4.

 gluten free
also nut free

Follow the nut-free recipe, but replace the flour with an equal quantity of gluten-free flour.

VARIATION Use soft dark brown sugar instead of granulated sugar to make darker, chewier biscuits. This will make a wetter dough, which you will need to drop in spoonfuls onto the baking sheets.

Gingerbread

This moist and sticky, lightly-spiced gingerbread is wonderfully versatile. You can serve it warm, without the icing, topped with whipped cream and a little scattered chopped crystallized ginger or with some ginger syrup poured over it. Thickly topped with the lemon icing, it looks very festive and makes an excellent tea-time treat, as well as being a winner in lunchboxes and at school fêtes.

 ## nut free

a little flavourless nut-free
  vegetable oil for greasing
280g (10oz) plain flour
½ tsp bicarbonate of soda
½ tsp salt
1 tbsp ground ginger
2 tsp ground cinnamon
1 tsp ground allspice
150g (5½oz) caster sugar
115g (4oz) butter, melted and
  cooled to room temperature
225g (8oz) molasses
250ml (8½fl oz) milk
1 egg, beaten

to serve
a little stem ginger in syrup
cream
or lemon glacé icing
250g (8½ oz) icing sugar
1½ tbsp lemon juice
1½ –2 tbsp water
to decorate
crystallized or stem ginger pieces
  (optional)

PREPARATION TIME 10 minutes
COOKING TIME 50–60 minutes
MAKES 1 slab cake

1 Preheat the oven to 180°C (350°F, gas 4).
2 Grease a 18 x 28cm (7 x 11in) shallow baking tin with oil and line with baking parchment.
3 Sift together into a bowl the dry ingredients: flour, bicarbonate of soda, salt, ginger, cinnamon, and allspice. Stir in the sugar.
4 Add the dry ingredients to the wet ingredients and mix to combine, but do not overmix.
5 Pour the gingerbread batter into the baking tin and smooth the top with a palette knife, if necessary.
6 Bake for 50–60 minutes, until the gingerbread springs back when pressed. Cool slightly then turn out onto a plate, if serving warm, or cool on a wire rack.
7 Either serve warm with whipped cream and a little chopped stem ginger in syrup, if liked, or when cool make the icing.
8 Sift the icing sugar into a bowl and add the lemon juice. Beat in enough water to form a thick, spreadable paste.
9 Spread the icing over the gingerbread and use a palette knife dipped in warm water to smooth if liked or let it drip attractively over the sides. Decorate with crystallized ginger, if liked.

 ## dairy free
also nut free

Follow the nut-free recipe, but substitute the butter with an equal quantity of dairy-free spread and the milk with an equal quantity of soya, oat, or rice milk.

 ## egg free
also nut free

Follow the nut-free recipe, but replace the egg with 1 tablespoon of potato flour plus 3 tablespoons of water. Add the potato flour to the dry ingredients in step 3 and the water to the wet ingredients in step 4.

 ## gluten free
also nut free

Follow the nut-free recipe, but replace the flour with an equal quantity of gluten-free flour mix or use rice flour instead – this gives a crumblier texture and a pleasant taste.

TIP If you are cutting the gingerbread into squares, then do this before icing it, as cutting the iced cake can crack the icing.

Fruity flapjacks

These sweet, golden squares are full of dried fruit and other good things. A great snack with a cup of tea or in the lunchbox, they keep your energy levels up without ruining your appetite. The millet version is closer to a deliciously crumbly shortbread than to the classic oat flapjack, and is a nice change whether or not you have to be gluten free.

   ## egg & nut free

100g (3½oz) butter or
  margarine plus extra for
  greasing
30g (1oz) demerara sugar
2 generous tbsp golden syrup
225g (8oz) rolled oats
½ tsp mixed spice
30g (1oz) sultanas
30g (1oz) raisins
30g (1oz) dried apricots,
  chopped

PREPARATION TIME 15 minutes
COOKING TIME 25 minutes
MAKES 16

 ## dairy free
also egg & nut free

Follow the recipe on the left, but substitute dairy-free spread for the butter or ordinary margarine.

gluten free
also egg & nut free

Follow the recipe on the left, but substitute millet or quinoa flakes for the oats.

1 Preheat the oven to 180°C (350°F, gas 4). Grease an 18 x 28cm (7 x 11in) baking tin.
2 Melt the butter or margarine with the sugar and syrup in a large saucepan.
3 Stir in all the remaining ingredients.
4 Transfer the mixture to the baking tin and press out firmly into the corners, using the back of a wet spoon. Bake in the centre of the oven for about 25 minutes or until a rich golden brown. Check after 20 minutes to ensure the edges are not getting too brown.
5 Leave to cool slightly then mark into 16 squares. Cool completely in the tin then remove and store in an airtight container.

BREADS & BAKING

Chocolate crinkle cookies

These are sophisticated little biscuits, rolled in a generous amount of icing sugar to create a snowy coating that cracks attractively and dramatically on cooking to reveal the sweet dark chocolate interior. Intended as an adult treat they turned out to be remarkably popular with children. They are quick and easy to make and need just half an hour to chill the dough.

  ## egg & nut free

45g (1½oz) granulated sugar
85g (3oz) self-raising flour
1 tsp bicarbonate of soda
30g (1oz) nut-free cocoa powder
55g (2oz) butter
2 tbsp golden syrup
45g (1½oz) icing sugar
  for coating

PREPARATION TIME 20 minutes
  plus chilling time
COOKING TIME 10–12 minutes
MAKES 16 small or 8 large cookies

1 Place the sugar in a medium bowl. Sift in the flour, bicarbonate of soda, and cocoa powder.

2 Add the butter and rub in with your fingers until the mixture has the consistency of breadcrumbs. Stir in the golden syrup and mix well. Draw the dough together with your hands to form a ball.

3 Divide the dough into 16 pieces for small biscuits or 8 for large biscuits. Chill them in the fridge for at least 30 minutes.

4 Preheat the oven to 180°C (350°F, gas 4). Line 2 baking sheets with baking parchment.

5 Roll each piece of dough into a ball and roll in the icing sugar, coating very thickly, before placing them on the lined baking sheets at least 4cm (1½in) apart, as they spread during baking.

6 Bake in the oven until attractively cracked on the top and still a little bit soft in the centre. Check the small biscuits after 10 minutes and the double-size biscuits after 12 minutes.

7 Allow the cookies to firm up on the baking sheet before transferring to a wire rack to cool. Store in an airtight container.
Pictured on next page ▶

 ## dairy free
also egg & nut free

Follow the recipe on the left, but use dairy-free spread instead of butter.

 ## gluten free
also egg & nut free

Follow the recipe on the left, but substitute an equal quantity of gluten-free self-raising flour for the flour and ensure that the bicarbonate of soda and cocoa powder are also gluten free.

TIP If you can't get self-raising gluten-free flour, convert gluten-free plain flour by adding 2 teaspoons of gluten-free baking powder.

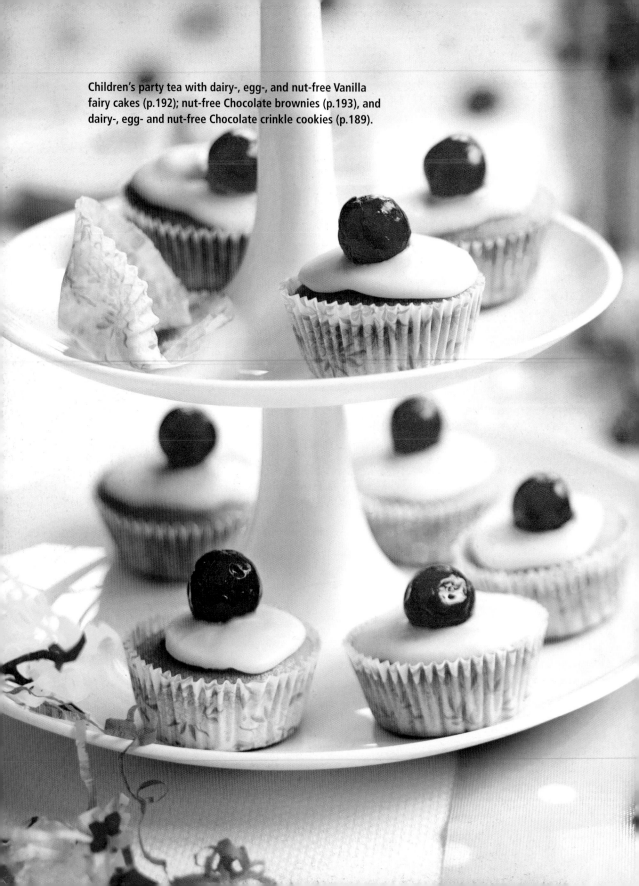

Children's party tea with dairy-, egg-, and nut-free Vanilla fairy cakes (p.192); nut-free Chocolate brownies (p.193), and dairy-, egg- and nut-free Chocolate crinkle cookies (p.189).

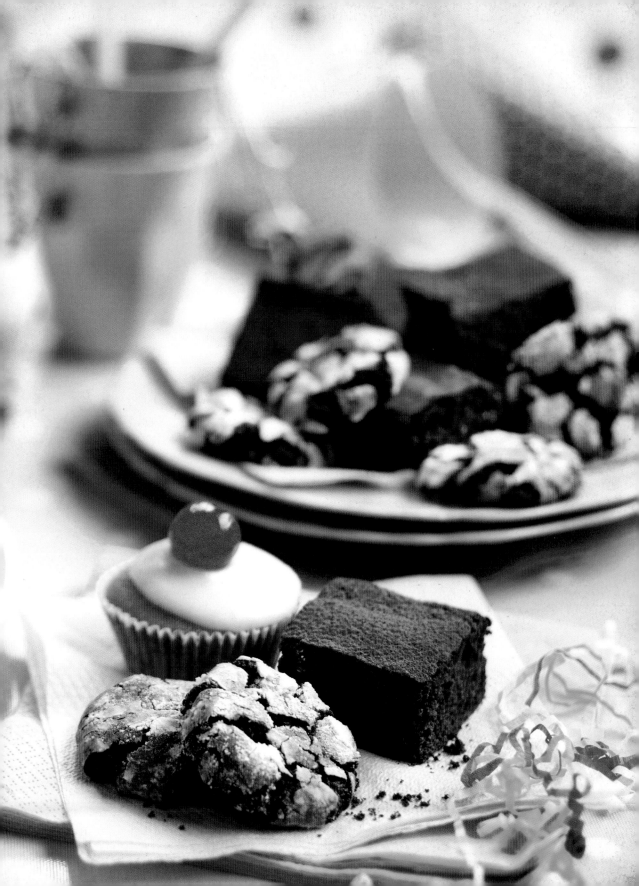

Vanilla fairy cakes

Vanilla fairy cakes are a childhood staple and a centrepiece at children's parties. They also figure in many children's first experiences of cooking at home or at school, which makes it a shame for those who can't join in because of food hypersensitivities. Here are versions – made easy for little hands – that make it possible for everyone to take part.

   dairy, egg & nut free

170g (6oz) plain flour
1 tbsp baking powder
pinch of salt
140g (5oz) soft light brown
  sugar
1 tsp vanilla extract
2 tbsp corn or other flavourless
  nut-free vegetable oil
1 tbsp white wine vinegar
240ml (8fl oz) water

PREPARATION TIME 15 minutes
COOKING TIME 20 minutes
MAKES 12

1 Preheat the oven to 180°C (350°F, gas 4). Line 12 sections of a tartlet tin or small muffin pan with paper fairy cake cases.
2 Sift the flour, baking powder, and salt into a bowl. Stir in the sugar.
3 Add the remaining ingredients and beat until you have a smooth, liquid batter.
4 Pour or ladle the batter into the cake cases, filling to just below the top of the case. Bake in the oven for about 20 minutes or until risen and firm to touch.
5 Transfer to a wire rack to cool.
◀ **Pictured on previous page**

TIP If you are making these with children, place the batter in a jug for easier pouring in step 4.

SERVING SUGGESTION For a children's party, decorate the cakes with icing and a glacé cherry on top. To make the glacé icing sift 200g (7oz) of icing sugar into a bowl. Add 2–2½ tablespoons of water and a few drops of food colouring, if liked, and mix to a thick, spreadable cream.

 gluten free
also nut free

3 eggs
140g (5oz) soft, light brown sugar
½ tsp vanilla extract
85g (3oz) butter or margarine,
  melted
85g (3oz) potato flour
85g (3oz) soya flour
2½ tsp gluten-free baking powder

• Preheat the oven to 180°C (350°F, gas 4). Line 12 sections of a tartlet tin or small muffin pan with fairy cake cases.
• Break the eggs into a bowl and add the sugar. Whisk with an electric or balloon whisk until thick and pale and the mixture leaves a trail when the whisk is lifted out of the batter.
• Whisking all the time, add the melted butter or margarine in a thin trickle.
• Sift the flours and baking powder over the surface. Fold in with a metal spoon, using a figure of eight motion.
• Spoon into the cake cases. Bake in the oven for 15–20 minutes, until risen and the centres spring back when lightly pressed.
• Transfer to a wire rack to cool.

Chocolate brownies

These are as brownies should be: rich, moist chocolatey squares with a distinctively cracked top. For extra interest, add a handful of raisins or sultanas to the mixture, or chopped walnuts, if you can eat them. Enjoy them at tea time or at any other time! My favourite is to eat them warm, for dessert, with the best vanilla ice cream I can find.

 nut free

85g (3oz) plain flour
1 tbsp nut-free cocoa powder
good pinch of salt
1 tsp baking powder
170g (6oz) soft light brown
  sugar
55g (2oz) butter or margarine
2 tbsp water
100g (3½oz) nut-free plain
  chocolate
1 tsp vanilla extract
2 large eggs, beaten

PREPARATION TIME 25 minutes
COOKING TIME 20 minutes
MAKES 15

1 Preheat the oven to 180°C (350°F, gas 4). Line an 18 x 28cm (7 x 11in) baking tin with baking parchment.
2 Sift the flour, cocoa powder, salt, and baking powder into a bowl.
3 Put the sugar, butter or margarine, water, chocolate, and vanilla in a saucepan and heat gently, stirring, until melted.
4 Pour into the flour mixture, add the eggs, and beat until smooth.
5 Transfer to the prepared tin and bake for about 20 minutes, until firm to the touch and slightly crusty on top.
6 Leave the brownies to cool for 10 minutes then mark into 15 squares. Cool completely before removing from the tin. Store in an airtight container.
◀ **Pictured on page 191**

 dairy free
also nut free

Follow the nut-free recipe, but make sure you use dairy-free margarine instead of butter or magarine and check that the plain chocolate is dairy free, too.

 egg free
also nut free

Follow the nut-free recipe to step 4 adding an extra ½ teaspoon of baking powder to the mix. At step 4, omit the eggs. Mix 15g (½oz) potato flour and 150ml (5fl oz) water in a small saucepan. Bring to the boil until just thickened and clear, stirring all the time. Remove from the heat. Beat the potato flour and water mixture into the flour mixture along with the melted ingredients. These egg-free brownies are even more moist and chewy than the others.

 gluten free
also nut free

Follow the nut-free recipe, but substitute gluten-free plain white flour for the ordinary flour and check that the baking powder and cocoa powder are gluten free, too.

Raspberry mallow crispies

Simple and inexpensive to make, these sticky cereal squares are a children's party treat – so they are just the thing whether your young guests have allergies or not. The puffed rice gives them an attractive honeycombed appearance. The dairy-free version is very useful for larger events as you can serve them to anyone with any of the Big Four allergies.

   gluten, egg & nut free

a little nut-free vegetable oil
  for greasing
115g (4oz) marshmallows
  (preferably pink and white)
55g (2oz) butter
4 tbsp raspberry jam
140g (5oz) puffed rice cereal

PREPARATION TIME 10 minutes
  plus chilling time
MAKES 24

 dairy free
also gluten, egg & nut free

Follow the recipe on the left, but substitute dairy-free spread for the butter.

1 Grease an 18 x 28cm (7 x 11in) shallow baking tin.
2 Put the marshmallows in a large saucepan with the butter and the jam. Heat gently, stirring all the time, until everything has melted. Then boil for 1 minute, stirring throughout.
3 Stir in the cereal fairly rapidly until thoroughly coated in the sticky mixture.
4 Transfer the mixture to the prepared tin; spread it right to the corners; then press down firmly using a wet palette knife or the back of a spoon. Use a knife to mark it into 24 squares. Leave the mixture until cold then chill it overnight to firm.
5 Store in an airtight container.

WATCH OUT FOR marshmallows that have been sweetened with maltodextrin or other sugars derived from barley, if you can't eat gluten. Some brands of marshmallow may contain egg. Check the puffed rice cereal for ingredients containing dairy or gluten, if need be.

Lemon syrup polenta cake

A fresh tasting gâteau, golden-brown on the outside and gloriously yellow on the inside, which can be served as a dessert or at tea time. It's lovely accompanied by fresh summer fruits, blackberries, or blueberries and, if you are feeling indulgent, some dollops of Chantilly topping (p.216), too. The lemon syrup is delightfully tangy, or try the rosemary syrup for something unusual and rather special.

 gluten free

for the cake
a little nut-free oil for greasing
140g (5oz) butter
140g (5oz) caster sugar
2 eggs, beaten
140g (5oz) ground almonds
1 tsp vanilla extract
85g (3oz) polenta or other
   cornmeal
½ tsp baking powder
¼ tsp salt
grated zest and juice of
   1 large lemon

for the syrup
4 tbsp lemon juice (juice of 2 lemons)
2 tbsp water
115g (4oz) icing sugar

PREPARATION TIME 15 minutes
COOKING TIME 1 hour
SERVES 8–10

1 Preheat the oven to 180°C (350°F, gas 4). Grease a deep 18cm (7in) round cake tin and line it with baking parchment.
2 Beat together the butter and sugar either with an electric whisk or a wooden spoon, until soft and fluffy.
3 Add in the eggs a little at a time, whisking well after each addition.
4 Add the ground almonds and vanilla extract. Sift the polenta, baking powder, and salt over. Add the lemon zest and juice and fold everything in gently with a metal spoon.
5 Transfer the cake mixture to the prepared tin and level the surface.
6 Bake for 1 hour or until risen, golden, and firm to touch. Remove the cake from the oven.
7 To make the syrup, gently heat together the lemon juice, water, and icing sugar in a small saucepan, stirring until the sugar has completely dissolved.
8 Stab the cake all over with a wooden cocktail stick, making the holes go almost to the base. Spoon the hot syrup over the cake – there is quite a lot but it all soaks in.
9 Leave the cake to cool completely in the tin before turning out and removing the baking parchment.

 dairy free
also gluten free

Follow the gluten-free recipe, but use dairy-free spread instead of butter.

 egg free
also gluten free

Follow the gluten-free recipe, but substitute 4 tablespoons of soured cream plus 2 tablespoons of potato flour blended with 2 tablespoons of water for the eggs. Increase the baking powder to 1 teaspoon.

 nut free
also gluten free

Follow the gluten-free recipe, but substitute gluten-free self-raising flour for the ground almonds and omit the baking powder. Use 3 eggs instead of 2 to keep the cake moist.

VARIATION An unusual variation is to use rosemary syrup. Heat together 4 tablespoons of water, 2 tablespoons of lemon juice, 85g (3oz) of caster sugar, and a sprig of rosemary until the sugar dissolves. Boil for 1 minute then leave to cool for 5 minutes. Strain the syrup over the cake. Decorate with fresh rosemary sprigs.

Chocolate layer cake

Ideal for celebrations and birthdays, this intensely flavoured chocolate cake, layered and topped with ganache or chocolate buttercream, is universally popular. The version pictured is egg, dairy, and nut free and is particularly impressive to anyone who knows how flat and disappointing some vegan concoctions can be. The secret is to bake the cake in two tins, split each one, sandwich the layers, and cover with icing.

   dairy, egg & nut free

for the cake
340g (12oz) plain flour
400g (14oz) caster sugar
1¾ tsp bicarbonate of soda
55g (2oz) nut-free cocoa
    powder
¼ tsp salt
450ml (15fl oz) unsweetened
    soya milk or water
100ml (3½fl oz) corn or other
    nut-free vegetable oil, plus
    extra for greasing
1½ tbsp white vinegar
1½ tsp vanilla extract

for the icing
a double quantity of ganache
    (p.200) or 1 quantity of chocolate
    buttercream icing (see right)
to decorate
    45g (1½oz) extra chocolate,
    shaved with a potato peeler,
    or a selection of fresh berries,
    if preferred

PREPARATION TIME 25 minutes
COOKING TIME 40 minutes
SERVES 10–12

1 Preheat the oven to 180°C (350°F, gas 4). Grease and line with baking parchment the bases of two deep 20cm (8in), round sandwich tins.
2 Sift together into a large bowl the flour, sugar, bicarbonate of soda, cocoa, and salt. In a separate bowl, mix together the liquid ingredients: the soya milk or water, oil, vinegar, and vanilla extract, and add to the flour mixture. Stir until smooth.
3 Divide the mixture between the prepared tins, and use a palette knife or spatula to spread evenly. Bake in the oven for about 40 minutes, until risen and firm to the touch.
4 Cool in the tins for 10 minutes then turn out onto a wire rack, remove the baking parchment and leave to cool completely. Slice each cake in half horizontally.
5 Meanwhile, make the ganache following step 7 of the recipe on page 200, or make chocolate buttercream icing.
6 Sandwich the cakes together using half the ganache or buttercream for the first three layers. Spread the remainder on the top and sides and rough up with a knife. Sprinkle with chocolate shavings or decorate with fresh berries.
Pictured opposite ▶

 gluten free

See overleaf for gluten-free recipe.

VARIATION For a lighter, more child-friendly icing make chocolate buttercream. Put 175g (6oz) dairy-free spread in a bowl and sift over 450g (1lb) icing sugar and 6 tablespoons of cocoa powder (nut free, if required). Add 2 teaspoons of vanilla extract. Gradually work into the spread with a wooden spoon then beat well until smooth and fluffy.
    If you don't need to avoid dairy products, use butter or ordinary margarine, increasing the quantity to 225g (8oz). You may need to add 4 teaspoons of water to give the correct soft consistency for spreading.

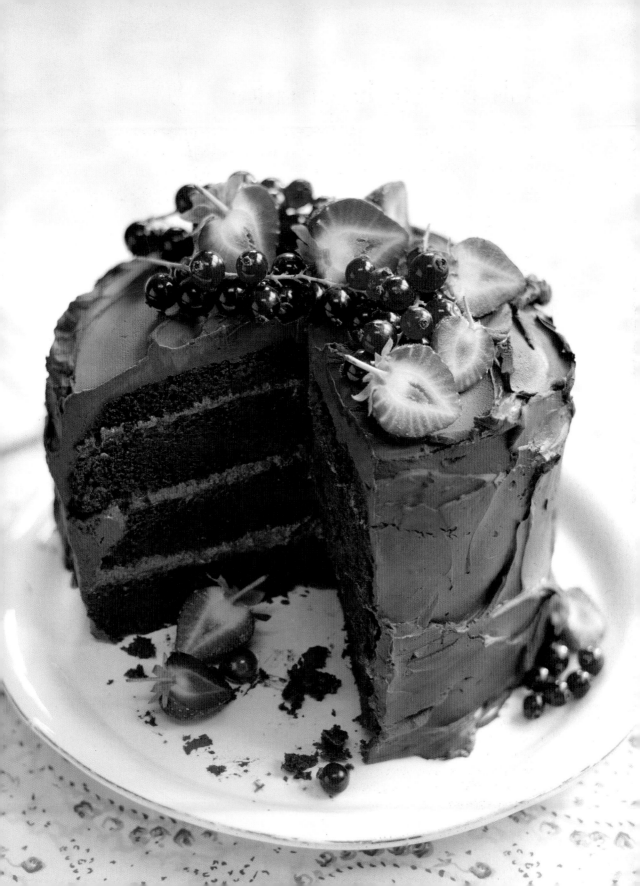

Chocolate layer cake continued

 gluten free

a little flavourless oil for greasing
6 eggs
340g (12oz) caster sugar
170g (6oz) butter or margarine, melted
½ tsp vanilla extract
200g (7oz) soya flour
125g (4½oz) potato flour

75g (2½oz) gluten-free cocoa powder
1½ tbsp gluten-free baking powder
2 tbsp milk

PREPARATION TIME 35 minutes
COOKING TIME 45 minutes
SERVES 10–12

1 Preheat the oven to 160°C (325°F, gas 3). Grease two deep 20cm (8in) round sandwich tins and line the bases with baking parchment.
2 Break the eggs into a bowl and add the sugar. Place the bowl over a pan of gently simmering water and whisk with an electric whisk until thick and pale and the mixture leaves a trail when the whisk is lifted out of the mixture – this will take several minutes.
3 Remove the bowl from the pan. Gradually add the melted butter or margarine in a thin trail, whisking all the time. Whisk in the vanilla extract.
4 Sift the flours, cocoa, and baking powder over the surface. Add the milk. Gently fold in with a metal spoon, using a figure of eight motion.
5 Divide the mixture between the prepared tins, and use a palette knife or spatula to spread evenly.
6 Bake in the oven for about 45 minutes, until risen and firm to the touch.
7 Cool in the tins for 10 minutes then turn out onto a wire rack, remove the baking parchment and leave to cool completely. Slice each cake in half horizontally.
8 Make a double quantity of ganache according to step 7 of the recipe on page 200 or make the buttercream icing on page 196. Sandwich the cakes together using half the frosting. Spread the remainder on the top and sides and rough up with a knife. Sprinkle with chocolate shavings or decorate with fresh berries.

WATCH OUT FOR intolerance to soya flour – if necessary, use gram or rice flour instead.

"If you need a super, fail-safe chocolate cake for any occasion, this is the one"

Rich fruit cake

This cake has a wonderful richness and flavour and is packed with goodness. The grated apple makes for an extra-moist texture, too. Sprinkle it with demerara sugar before baking for a lovely crunchy topping. If you want to adapt your own recipes, fruit cakes are a good place to start. Use the cooking tips in Substituting ingredients (p.48) or the versions below for inspiration.

nut free

a little nut-free vegetable oil for greasing
1 eating apple, grated, including the skin
170g (6oz) softened butter or margarine
170g (6oz) soft, light brown sugar
3 eggs
225g (8oz) plain flour
pinch of salt

1½ tsp baking powder
1½ tsp ground mixed spice
225g (8oz) mixed dried fruit
55g (2oz) glacé cherries, halved
1 tbsp demerara sugar

PREPARATION TIME 10 minutes
COOKING TIME 1½–1¾ hours
SERVES 8–10

1 Preheat the oven to 160°C (325°F, gas 3). Grease and line with baking parchment a high-sided 18cm (7in) cake tin.
2 Beat the apple with the butter or margarine and the soft brown sugar until light and fluffy.
3 Beat in the eggs, one at a time, beating well after each addition (this mixture will curdle a bit).
4 Sift the flour, salt, baking powder, and spice over the surface. Fold in with a metal spoon, then fold in the mixed dried fruit and cherries.
5 Transfer the mixture to the prepared tin and level the surface. Sprinkle with the demerara sugar.
6 Bake in the oven until the cake is richly browned, firm to the touch and a skewer inserted in the centre comes out clean (1½–1¾ hours). Leave to cool in the tin for 10 minutes, then turn out onto a wire rack, remove the baking parchment and leave to cool completely. This cake keeps well stored in an airtight container.

TIP Fruit cakes are amongst the easiest of cake recipes to adapt to egg free. Just replace each egg with 1 tablespoon of potato flour mixed with 3 tablespoons of water in your favourite fruit cake recipes.

dairy free
also nut free

Follow the nut-free recipe, but substitute dairy-free spread for the butter or margarine.

egg free
also nut free

Follow the nut-free recipe, but omit the eggs in step 3 and add 3 tablespoons of flavourless nut-free vegetable oil and 1 tablespoon of potato flour mixed with 3 tablespoons of water as an egg substitute. Increase the baking powder to 2 teaspoons and add with the other dry ingredients in step 4.

gluten free
also nut free

Follow the nut-free recipe, but for the plain flour substitute an equal quantity of gluten-free flour or 115g (4oz) brown rice flour and 115g (4oz) soya flour and check the baking powder is gluten free, too.

Dark chocolate torte

This rich chocolate torte, a close relation of the famous Sachertorte, is an elegant dark chocolate sponge, apricot-glazed and iced with bittersweet chocolate. A wonderfully decadent dessert for a dinner party, either on its own or with unsweetened lightly whipped or pouring cream (or non-dairy alternative). If possible, use chocolate with 70 per cent cocoa solids to get the true richness.

 gluten free

for the torte
170g (6oz) plain chocolate with 70 per cent cocoa solids
115g (4oz) unsalted butter plus a little extra for greasing
115g (4oz) icing sugar, sifted
150g (5½oz) ground almonds
5 eggs, separated
1 tbsp apricot jam

for the ganache
115g (4oz) plain chocolate with 70 per cent cocoa solids
120ml (4fl oz) double cream

PREPARATION TIME 45 minutes
COOKING TIME 30 minutes
SERVES 8–10

1 Preheat the oven to 190°C (375°F, gas 5). Grease a 20cm (8in) springform tin and line the base with baking parchment.

2 Break up the chocolate and place it in a bowl. Stand the bowl over a pan of simmering water and stir until the chocolate has melted. Alternatively, heat briefly in the microwave.

3 In a separate bowl, beat together the butter and icing sugar until light and fluffy. Beat in the nuts, egg yolks, and chocolate.

4 Whisk the egg whites until stiff and fold in with a metal spoon.

5 Transfer to the prepared tin and smooth the surface. Bake in the oven until firm to the touch (about 30 minutes). Leave to cool in the tin for 10 minutes then remove the tin and transfer the torte to a wire rack to cool completely.

6 Warm the jam in a small saucepan and sieve.

7 Make the ganache. Break up the chocolate and place it in a separate pan with the cream. Heat gently, stirring all the time with a wooden spoon until thick. Leave to cool slightly until it is a thick, coating consistency.

8 Transfer the torte to a serving plate. Spread the top with the warmed jam. Spoon the ganache over, spreading it out with a palette knife so it coats the top and sides of the torte completely. Wipe the edge of the plate to clean up any excess chocolate. Leave to set but do not chill.

TIP I like to coat the torte on its plate as it saves disturbing it once it is finished, but if you prefer, you can coat the torte when it's on the cooling rack then transfer it to a plate when set.

 dairy free
also gluten free

Follow the gluten-free recipe, but substitute dairy-free spread for the butter in the torte. For the ganache, increase the chocolate to 140g (5oz) and use 5 tablespoons of soya cream alternative in place of the double cream. Use dairy-free chocolate. If you can't tolerate soya, make a chocolate glacé icing. Melt very gently 85g (3oz) chocolate with 15g (½oz) dairy-free spread and 3 tablespoons of water. Gradually beat in 225g (8oz) sifted icing sugar.

 egg free
also gluten free

Follow the gluten-free recipe, but omit the egg yolks and add 2 teaspoons of baking powder with the ground almonds. Whisk 3 tablespoons of potato flour with 1 teaspoon of xanthan gum and 150ml (5fl oz) water until white and softly peaked and use in place of egg whites.

 nut free
also gluten free

Follow the gluten-free recipe, but substitute 100g (3½oz) fine nut-free breadcrumbs or nut-free sponge cake crumbs for the ground almonds.

Peach-topped cheesecake

This is a lovely deli-style cheesecake with a glossy fruit topping. It is simple to make, with no baking involved and lends itself well to variations, so change the biscuit base and topping to taste. Try coconut biscuits with a mango nectar topping, or a gingernut base with a berry topping – there are many combinations, just be sure to use the thick "nectar" style of juice.

  egg & nut free

for the base
170g (6oz) digestive biscuits
   (nut free and egg free)
75g (2½oz) butter, melted plus
   a little extra for greasing

for the filling
1 tbsp powdered gelatine
250ml (8½fl oz) peach nectar
115g (4oz) caster sugar
380g (13oz) cream cheese
1 vanilla pod
1 tbsp lemon juice
250ml (8½fl oz) double cream

for the peach topping
1 tbsp cornflour
1 tbsp caster sugar
2 tsp lemon juice
250ml (8½fl oz) peach nectar

PREPARATION TIME 20 minutes
   plus chilling time
SERVES 6–8

1 Grease a 20cm (8in) springform tin and line the base with baking parchment. In a food processor, crush the biscuits to crumbs then add the melted butter and process again briefly to combine. Press into the prepared tin and chill for 30 minutes.

2 Make the filling. Sprinkle the gelatine over 5 tablespoons of the peach nectar in a small bowl. Stir well. Leave to soften for 5 minutes then stand the bowl in a pan of gently simmering water and stir until dissolved completely. Stir in the remaining peach nectar. Leave to cool.

3 Place the sugar and cream cheese in a large bowl and beat together using an electric whisk. Split the vanilla pod lengthways and scrape its contents into the bowl. Pour in the lemon juice and the peach nectar and gelatine mixture, and whisk well to combine. Lightly whip the cream until softly peaking and fold in with a metal spoon. Spoon the filling over the biscuit base and chill overnight, or for at least 4 hours until set.

4 Make the peach topping. Place the cornflour and sugar in a small saucepan. Blend in the lemon juice then the nectar and stir well. Bring to the boil and boil for 1 minute, stirring constantly, until thickened and smooth. Remove immediately from the heat. Allow to cool slightly before spreading carefully over the cheesecake.

5 Chill again before serving.

 dairy free
also egg & nut free

Follow the recipe on the left, but replace the butter used in the base with an equal quantity of dairy-free spread. Increase the gelatine from 1 to 1½ tablespoons. Replace the cream cheese with an equal quantity of soya cream cheese alternative and the double cream with an equal quantity of soya cream alternative (which will not whip as thickly as dairy cream). For a firmer cheesecake, increase the gelatine to 2 tablespoons.

 gluten free
also egg & nut free

Follow the recipe on the left, making sure that the biscuits used in the base are gluten free.

TIP This is not a cheesecake to leave out on a hot day – it will turn into a fruit mousse cake! Make sure you chill it well to set before serving.

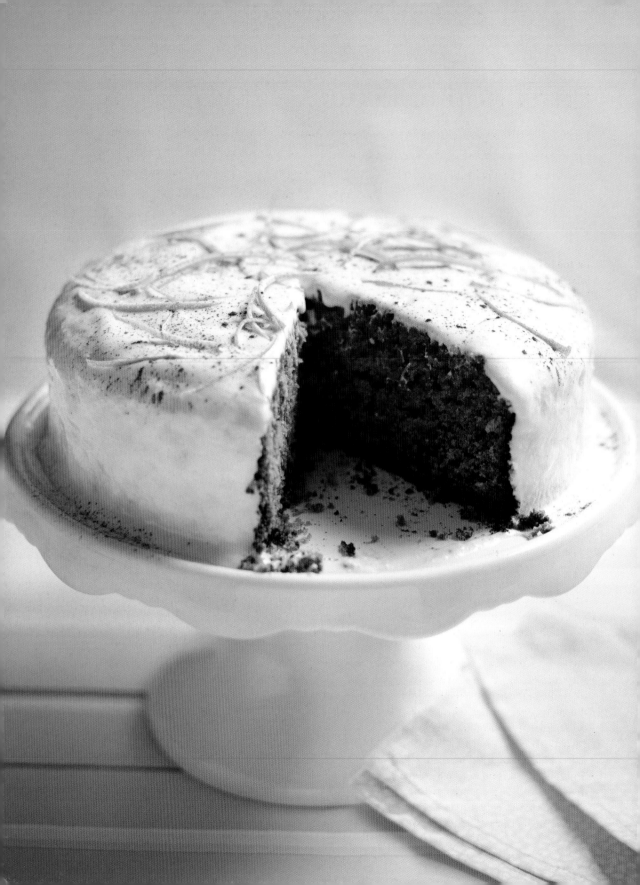

Carrot cake

A luxurious carrot cake as celebratory as any fruit cake. This one is lightly spiced with nutmeg, allspice, and cinnamon and crammed full of luscious ingredients from pineapple and coconut to brown sugar and sultanas. Using both puréed and raw carrots makes the cake delectably moist; you can also use pine nuts instead of the usual walnuts. Delicious with or without its classic vanilla cream cheese icing.

 nut free

for the cake
450g (1lb) self-raising flour
2 tsp baking powder
2 tsp ground cinnamon
¼ tsp grated nutmeg
½ tsp ground allspice
225g (8oz) soft dark brown sugar
250ml (8½fl oz) flavourless nut-free vegetable oil
3 eggs, lightly beaten
225g (8oz) cooked carrots, cooled and puréed
115g (4oz) grated raw carrot
115g (4oz) pine nuts, lightly toasted and roughly chopped, if tolerated (optional)
115g (4oz) sultanas

55g (2oz) desiccated coconut, if tolerated
55g (2oz) canned crushed pineapple, drained
finely grated zest of 1 orange

for the icing
250g (8½oz) cream cheese
500g (1lb 2oz) icing sugar
180g (6½oz) unsalted butter
1 tsp vanilla extract

to decorate
finely pared zest of 1 orange
sprinkling of ground cinnamon

PREPARATION TIME 15 minutes
COOKING TIME 1¼ – 1½ hours
SERVES 12

1 Preheat the oven to 180°C (350°F, gas 4). Line a 23cm (9in) springform tin with baking parchment.

2 Sift together the flour, baking powder, cinnamon, nutmeg, and allspice. Add the brown sugar and mix well.

3 Add the oil, beaten eggs, carrot purée, raw carrot, pine nuts (if used), sultanas, coconut, pineapple, and orange zest. Mix well. It should be a very thick, wet dough. Alternatively, combine all the ingredients in a food processor and mix thoroughly.

4 Spoon the mixture into the prepared tin. Place in the oven and bake until a skewer inserted in the centre comes out clean and the edges pull away from the sides of the tin, about 1¼–1½ hours.

5 Cool the cake in the tin for 15 minutes, then release the cake onto a wire rack, remove the paper, and leave to cool. The top may look cracked but it will be covered by the icing.

6 To make the icing, put all the ingredients into a food processor and blend until smooth, about 1 minute. Smooth over the top and sides of the cold cake. To decorate, sprinkle with orange zest and cinnamon. Chill, if necessary, to firm up the icing.

 dairy free
also nut free

The cake is dairy free. For the icing (pictured opposite), use soya-based cream cheese alternative for the cream cheese and dairy-free spread for the butter. If necessary, add a little more icing sugar to the icing. This version needs to be refrigerated as the icing will soften if left too long at room temperature.

 egg free
also nut free

Prepare as for the recipe on the left, but increase the baking powder to 2 tablespoons. Add the juice of the orange as well as the zest and substitute 3 tablespoons of potato flour, mixed with 6 tablespoons of water, for the eggs.

◀ Pictured opposite
With a dairy-free topping, it is also suitable for vegans.

 gluten free
also nut free

Prepare as for the recipe on the left, but use gluten-free plain white flour for the self-raising flour and increase the baking powder to 3 tablespoons (make sure it is gluten free).

Fresh fruit & cream gâteau

This is a party dessert to delight friends and family – towering layers of vanilla sponge, sandwiched with sweetened whipped cream, nectarines and figs. You can use any soft, seasonal fruit – berries work particularly well. As with the Chocolate layer cake (p.196), you bake it in two tins, then split the layers, fill, layer and top it. And yes, that is the egg-free version in the picture!

  ## egg & nut free

for the cake
400g (14oz) plain flour
400g (14oz) caster sugar
1¾ tsp bicarbonate of soda
¼ tsp salt
100ml (3½fl oz) flavourless nut free oil, plus a little extra for greasing
1½ tbsp white vinegar
2 tsp vanilla extract
450ml (15fl oz) milk

for the filling and topping
360ml (12fl oz) double cream
2 tbsp icing sugar, plus extra for dusting
3 large ripe peaches, stoned and sliced
1 ripe fig, quartered

PREPARATION TIME 35 minutes
COOKING TIME 40 minutes
SERVES 10–12

1 Preheat the oven to 180°C (350°F, gas 4). Grease two 20cm (8in) deep sandwich tins and line the bases with baking parchment.
2 Sift together into a large bowl the flour, caster sugar, bicarbonate of soda, and salt. In a separate bowl mix together the oil, vinegar, vanilla extract, and milk and add to the flour mixture. Stir until smooth.
3 Divide the mixture between the prepared tins (it will be quite runny). Bake in the oven until risen and firm to the touch (about 40 minutes).
4 Cool in the tins for 10 minutes then turn out onto a wire rack, remove the baking parchment and leave to cool completely.
5 Make the filling and topping. Whip the cream with the icing sugar until softly peaking.
6 Select about a third of the best-looking peach slices and reserve for decoration.
7 Split each cake in half horizontally. Put one piece on a serving plate. Top with a quarter of the cream then a third of the peaches not reserved for decoration. Repeat the layers then top with the last piece of cake and smother with the remaining cream. Decorate with the reserved peach slices and figs. Chill until ready to serve. Dust with a little icing sugar, if liked, just before serving.
Pictured opposite ▶

 ## dairy free
also egg & nut free

Follow the recipe on the left, but use soya, rice, or oat milk instead of the cow's milk. For the filling and topping use 1½ quantities of dairy-free Chantilly topping (p.216) in place of the whipped cream and icing sugar.

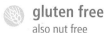 ## gluten free
also nut free

See overleaf for gluten-free recipe.

VARIATION Try using other fruit such as raspberries and nectarines for the filling and decoration. *Physalis* (Cape gooseberries) make a pretty garnish.

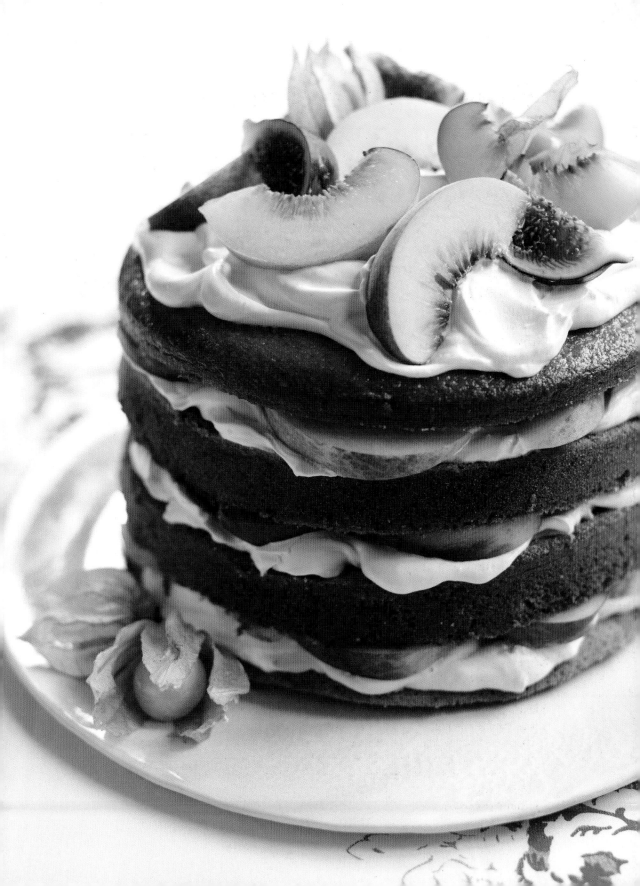

Fresh fruit & cream gâteau continued

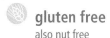 **gluten free**
also nut free

for the cake
a little flavourless nut-free oil
   for greasing
6 eggs
340g (12oz) caster sugar
170g (6oz) butter or margarine,
   melted
½ tsp vanilla extract
225g (8oz) soya flour
170g (6oz) potato flour
1½ tbsp gluten-free baking
   powder
2 tbsp milk

PREPARATION TIME 35 minutes
COOKING TIME 45 minutes
SERVES 10–12

1 Preheat the oven to 160°C (325°F, gas 3). Grease two 20cm (8in) deep sandwich tins and line the bases with baking parchment.

2 Break the eggs into a heatproof bowl and add the sugar. Place the bowl over a pan of gently simmering water and whisk with an electric whisk until thick and pale and the mixture leaves a trail when the whisk is lifted out – this will take several minutes.

3 Remove the bowl from the pan. Gradually add in the melted butter or margarine in a thin trail, whisking all the time. Whisk in the vanilla extract.

4 Sift the flours and baking powder over the surface. Add the milk. Gently fold in with a metal spoon, using a figure of eight motion.

5 Divide the mixture between the prepared tins and level the surfaces. Bake in the oven until risen and firm to the touch (about 45 minutes).

6 Cool in the tins for 10 minutes then turn out onto a wire rack, remove the baking parchment, and leave to cool completely.

7 Make the filling and topping as described on page 204. Split the cakes, sandwich them together, and decorate.

8 Chill until ready to serve. Dust with a little icing sugar, if liked, just before serving.

Chocolate truffles

This is more one for the grown ups with its slightly sophisticated dark chocolate taste. Truffles are a delightful way to finish a meal. Serve on a pretty dish or, if you can get petit four papers (like mini muffin cases) to put them in, so much the better. Wrapped in coloured or glittery paper, they make excellent presents, too – you can choose a liqueur to suit the occasion.

   egg, gluten & nut free

225g (8oz) plain chocolate with at least 70 per cent cocoa solids, nut-free and/or gluten-free, if necessary
125ml (4½fl oz) double cream
1 tbsp liqueur of choice, such as Grand Marnier or brandy (optional)
55g (2oz) icing sugar, sifted
30g (1oz) cocoa powder, nut-free and/or gluten-free, if necessary

PREPARATION TIME 15–20 minutes
COOKING TIME 5 minutes
MAKES 20 truffles

1 Chop the chocolate into 5mm (¼in) pieces. Place the pieces in a heatproof bowl.
2 Heat the cream in a saucepan to just below boiling point and pour onto the chocolate pieces. Leave for 5 minutes.
3 Use an electric whisk to whisk the chocolate and cream together until there are no lumps. Whisk in the liqueur, if using, and the icing sugar. Leave the mixture to cool then chill until it is beginning to firm.
4 Use a dessertspoon to scoop out the truffle mixture. Roll the mixture in the palm of your hands into 2cm (¾in) balls. Roll each one carefully in cocoa powder. Place on a plate or in petit four paper cases. Chill until firm.

TIP I tend to use clear liqueurs rather than creamy ones as they have a more intense flavour.

 dairy free
also egg, gluten & nut free

Follow the recipe on the left, but ensure the chocolate is dairy free. Use a soya cream alternative for the double cream and if you are using a liqueur make sure it is dairy free.

WATCH OUT FOR liqueurs that contain ingredients to be avoided. Avoid amaretto and nut-containing spirits for the nut-free version; grain-based liqueurs, such as whisky and vodka, if making gluten-free truffles; cream-based concoctions, such as Baileys, if making dairy-free truffles; and in the unlikely event you are going to put Advocaat into your chocolate truffles, please don't serve them to egg-allergics.

Béchamel sauce

The classic French béchamel sauce is a base ingredient for many recipes from Lasagne al forno (p.136) to Moussaka (p.128), and for making savoury Crêpes (p.162). It is worth taking the trouble to make it well; infusing the cloves and vegetables in the milk makes a real difference to the taste. It keeps well in the fridge, so make double the quantity if you need to.

  ## egg & nut free

450ml (15fl oz) milk
1 onion, peeled, halved, and
    studded with two whole cloves
6 peppercorns
4 parsley stalks
45g (1½oz) butter
30g (1oz) plain flour
2 tbsp single cream
salt and freshly ground black
    pepper

PREPARATION TIME 20 minutes
COOKING TIME 10–15 minutes
    plus 20 minutes to infuse
SERVES 4–6

1 Place the milk, clove-studded onion, peppercorns, and parsley stalks in a saucepan. Bring to the boil, simmer for 10 minutes and remove from the heat. Leave to infuse for 20 minutes before straining the milk back into a saucepan and discarding the vegetables.

2 Melt the butter on a low heat in a separate saucepan. Add the flour. Mix well and cook for about 2 minutes, taking care not to let the butter and flour mixture brown. Bring the infused milk to a simmer.

3 Keeping the flour and butter mixture on a low heat, add in the milk gradually, using a whisk to ensure there are no lumps. When all the milk has been incorporated, simmer the sauce on a very low heat for 8–10 minutes to get rid of any lingering floury taste, stirring constantly with a wooden spoon.

4 Stir in the cream. Season to taste with salt and pepper. If keeping for later, cover with a circle of wet greaseproof paper.

TIPS You can make a quick basic white sauce by omitting step 1 and adding a sachet of bouquet garni to the pan in step 3 before simmering the sauce. If a thinner pouring sauce is needed, add more warmed milk or stock in step 3.

 ## dairy free
also egg & nut free

Follow the recipe on the left, but use non-dairy spread instead of the butter; soya, rice, or oat milk in place of the cow's milk; and use soya cream alternative instead of the cream.

 ## gluten free
also egg & nut free

Follow the recipe on the left, but use 30g (1oz) of a gluten-free flour mix or a half-and-half mix of rice flour and cornflour.

Roast garlic tofu aïoli

I know I've included recipes for classic mayonnaise but this aïoli, safe for all of the "Big Four" allergies, was just too good to leave out. Use in the same way you would a garlicky, flavoursome sauce or mayonnaise – in sandwiches, dips, on roasted vegetables, or stirred into soups. Or use the roast garlic purée on its own as a delicious topping for Crostini (pp.72–73).

    dairy, egg, gluten & nut free

for the roast garlic purée
4 heads of garlic
100ml (3½fl oz) olive oil or
  vegetable/chicken stock
1 tsp fresh thyme (optional)
1 bay leaf (optional)
for the roast garlic tofu aïoli
¼ quantity roast garlic purée
  (see above)
400g (14oz) firm silken tofu
2 tbsp light (sweet) miso paste
120ml (4fl oz) lemon juice
1–2 tbsp water or olive oil
  to thin
salt and freshly ground black
  pepper to taste

PREPARATION TIME 5 minutes plus
  1–1½ hours for roasting the garlic
MAKES 550ml (18fl oz)

TIPS The aïoli has a slightly softer texture, with less hold to it than mayonnaise made with eggs.

If using olive oil for roasting the garlic, keep it to use as garlic-flavoured oil for roasting potatoes or other vegetables.

WATCH OUT FOR stock cubes, which may contain traces of dairy or gluten, if you're cooking for people with severe dairy or gluten sensitivities.

1 Preheat the oven to 180°C (350°F, gas 4).
2 To make the garlic purée, slice off the top 1 cm (½ in) of the garlic heads and discard.
3 Pack the garlic heads snugly in a small ovenproof dish, scatter over the thyme, and tuck in the bay leaf, if using. Pour over the oil or stock.
4 Cover tightly and put in the oven.
5 Bake for 1–1½ hours or until the heads are soft.
6 Remove from the oven and leave to cool.
7 Squeeze the garlic cloves from their skins and process to a purée in a food processor. At this stage, the garlic purée can be stored, covered, in the refrigerator for up to a week.
8 To make the roast garlic tofu aïoli, process the garlic purée, tofu, miso paste, and lemon juice to mayonnaise consistency in a food processor. If necessary, use water or olive oil to thin to the desired consistency.
9 Season to taste with salt and pepper.

Mayonnaise

It seemed a good idea to give a recipe for mayonnaise, as many commercial brands contain dairy, gluten, and even nuts. Naturally a home-made one doesn't. There's a super egg-free version too.

   dairy, gluten & nut free

1 egg
1 tsp Dijon mustard
¼ tsp salt
5 tbsp olive oil
5 tbsp nut-free
  vegetable oil

1 tsp lemon juice
1 tsp white wine vinegar

PREPARATION TIME 10 minutes
MAKES about 260ml (9fl oz)

1 Break the egg into a food processor. Add the mustard and salt. Run the machine briefly to mix.

2 Measure the oils in a measuring jug. With the machine running, trickle the oil in a thin, gradual stream. It will be runny at first then will thicken. When about three-quarters of the oil is added, add the lemon juice and vinegar and then add the remaining oil in a slightly faster stream. Taste and add a little more salt, if liked.

3 Store in an airtight container in the fridge for up to 3 days. Use as required.

 egg free

also dairy, gluten & nut free

2 tbsp potato flour
½ tsp xanthan gum
4 tbsp water
¼ tsp Dijon mustard
120ml (4fl oz) olive oil
1 tbsp lemon juice
1 tsp white wine vinegar
½ tsp caster sugar
salt and white pepper

Mix the potato flour, gum, and water in a food processor until white and peaking. Beat in the mustard. Now follow the recipe on the left from step 2, adding the sugar and seasoning with the lemon juice and vinegar.

Vietnamese dipping sauce

This indispensable seasoning and dipping sauce can be found on every table in Vietnam – its tangy sour-sweet flavour is addictive. Thai cuisine has a similar one, often garnished with fresh green herbs.

    dairy, egg, gluten & nut free

2 tbsp fresh lime juice
2 tbsp sugar (palm sugar in preference)
4 tbsp rice vinegar
4 tbsp Thai fish sauce
2 garlic cloves, crushed

½ red chilli, deseeded and finely chopped

PREPARATION TIME 5 minutes
MAKES about 175ml (6fl oz)

1 Place all the ingredients in a food processor and process for 30–45 seconds. If a foamy head forms on top don't worry, just pour the sauce out and discard the foam.

2 Serve in small open bowls as a dipping sauce.

VARIATION To create an attractive oriental pickle, peel and julienne a carrot and ½ a daikon or mouli (white radish) and mix with the dipping sauce.

WATCH OUT FOR chillies, as some people can't tolerate them.

SAUCES, DRESSINGS & ACCOMPANIMENTS

Pesto

The famous Genoese basil and pine nut sauce has many uses. Serve with pasta, stirred into rice salads, or in sandwiches. It works just as well without cheese.

   egg, gluten & nut free

50g (1¾oz) fresh basil leaves
45g (1½oz) pine nuts
2 garlic cloves, crushed
25g (scant 1oz) Parmesan, grated
240ml (8fl oz) extra virgin
  olive oil
salt and pepper to season

PREPARATION TIME 10 minutes
MAKES about 340g (12oz)

1 In a food processor, process the basil leaves, pine nuts, garlic, and Parmesan for about 30 seconds to form a rough paste.
2 Add the oil in a thin stream through the top or funnel with the food processor still running. You should have a thick paste. If it seems too dry, add 1–2 tablespoons more oil. Season to taste.

 dairy free
also egg, gluten & nut free

Follow the recipe on the left, but substitute the Parmesan with an equal quantity of dairy-free cheese or omit altogether for cheeseless pesto as shown on page 172 (with focaccia).

WATCH OUT FOR pine nuts, which are classified as a seed rather than a nut. Most people allergic to tree nuts and peanuts can eat pine nuts, but check before serving to them.

Red pepper dip

This dip is based on the Syrian-Turkish speciality *Muhammara*. Some people prefer it thick and paste-like; others prefer a dipping consistency. Serve with flatbreads, salad, vegetables, or as a sauce for grilled meats.

  dairy & egg free

3 red peppers, deseeded
2 tbsp nut-free oil for roasting
1 small chilli, deseeded
1 slice of bread (45g/1½oz)
85g (3oz) shelled walnuts
½ clove of garlic, peeled
1½ tbsp pomegranate molasses
2 tsp lemon juice
½–1 tsp salt

½ tsp ground cumin
5 tbsp olive oil
water to thin (optional)
1 tbsp finely chopped fresh parsley
  to garnish

PREPARATION TIME 5 minutes plus
  cooking time for peppers
SERVES 6

1 Preheat the oven to 180°C (350°F, gas 4). Roast the peppers in the oil for 40 minutes, until they are soft.
2 In a food processor, blend the peppers and the oil they were roasted in with the chilli, bread, walnuts, garlic, pomegranate molasses, lemon juice, salt, cumin, and olive oil until smooth.
3 Thin with water if required and garnish with parsley.

 nut free
also dairy & egg free

Follow the recipe on the left, but use toasted pine nuts instead of walnuts (but see warning in recipe above).

 gluten free
also dairy & egg free

Follow the recipe on the left, but use an equal quantity of gluten-free bread.

WATCH OUT FOR chillies, as some people can't tolerate them.

Asian slaw

This is coleslaw with a South-East Asian twist. Shredded cabbage and carrot is dressed with a tangy sweet and sour sauce and garnished with mint. The Vietnamese love it with grilled or poached chicken, either as a street café snack or made at home. For canapés, try a couple of spoonfuls heaped onto Japanese rice crackers, topped with a coriander sprig. It is pictured on page 125 with Vietnamese beef stew.

   dairy, egg, gluten & nut free

for the dressing
1 tbsp rice vinegar
2 tbsp caster or palm sugar
3 tbsp fresh lime juice
2 garlic cloves, crushed
½ red chilli, deseeded,
  and finely chopped
3 tbsp Thai fish sauce
4 tbsp flavourless nut-free oil
freshly ground black pepper
for the salad
200g (7oz) Chinese or small hard
  white cabbage, shredded

85g (3oz) carrots, grated or ribboned
  (with a potato peeler)
2 spring onions, thinly sliced
3 tbsp chopped fresh mint leaves
coriander sprigs to garnish (optional)

PREPARATION TIME 10 minutes
SERVES 4 as a side dish

1 In a food processor, process the rice vinegar, sugar, lime juice, garlic, chilli, and fish sauce for 30 seconds or until the sugar is dissolved. Add the oil and black pepper and process briefly to combine.

2 Just before serving, combine the cabbage and carrot in a bowl, pour over the dressing and mix well. Stir in the spring onions and chopped mint leaves and garnish with coriander if using.

SERVING SUGGESTIONS For a light lunch or supper, top Asian slaw with strips of grilled chicken and sprinkle with sesame seeds (if tolerated). Serve with French bread (pp.170–171).
  Serve on rice or prawn crackers as a pre-dinner canapé or as a side salad with Vietnamese beef stew (p.124) or any oriental-style braised or grilled meat.

WATCH OUT FOR chilli as some people can't tolerate it.

"This piquant, fresh-tasting salad is perfect for the dark days of winter"

Raita

Raita is a cooling south Asian condiment based on yogurt and is usually served alongside spicy dishes. This one has cucumber and cumin seeds and works well with grilled meats, fish, and curries.

   egg, gluten & nut free

2 tsp cumin seeds
10cm (4in) piece cucumber, peeled and finely diced
300ml (10fl oz) plain or Greek-style yogurt
salt and freshly ground black pepper

PREPARATION TIME 10 minutes
SERVES 4–6

1 Toast the cumin seeds in a dry heavy-based frying pan over a moderate heat for about 2 minutes, until they release their fragrance. Tip out of the pan onto a plate to prevent further cooking and leave to cool.
2 Mix the cucumber and yogurt together in a small bowl and season with salt and pepper. Sprinkle the cumin seeds on top.

 dairy free
also egg, gluten & nut free

Follow the recipe on the left, but substitute soya yogurt alternative for the cow's milk yogurt.

SERVING SUGGESTION Serve with Tandoori fish (p.98).

Tarragon dressing

This is a simple, creamy dressing that works really well on a salad, served with chicken, fish, or vegetables. I particularly like it on a chicken and avocado salad with baby spinach leaves.

   egg, gluten & nut free

6 tbsp olive oil
1 garlic clove, crushed (optional)
2 tsp caster sugar
finely grated zest and juice of 1 lemon
4 tbsp single cream
3 tbsp chopped fresh tarragon

good pinch of salt
good grinding of freshly ground black pepper

PREPARATION TIME 10 minutes plus chilling time
MAKES about 200ml (7fl oz)

1 Put all the ingredients in a clean, screw-topped jar.
2 Shake vigorously until thoroughly blended. Chill for at least 1 hour to allow the flavours to develop. Use as required. The dressing will keep in the fridge for up to 1 week.

 dairy free
also egg, gluten & nut free

Follow the recipe on the left, but substitute soya cream alternative for single cream.

Chestnut stuffing

Rich, flavourful, and traditional, creamy chestnut stuffing is perfect for a festive roast bird, as it complements but doesn't overpower the meal. Chestnuts are botanically nuts, but most people with nut allergies can tolerate them. If you already know you can eat chestnuts, you can continue doing so. If you can't or are not sure, use the variation at the bottom of the recipe.

  ### egg & nut free

115g (4oz) cooked chestnuts, peeled (if tolerated)
170g (6oz) pork sausage meat
55g (2oz) fresh white breadcrumbs
2 shallots or 1 small onion, very finely chopped
2 tbsp chopped fresh parsley
½ tsp salt
good grating of nutmeg
freshly ground black pepper
30g (1oz) butter, melted
2–3 tbsp single cream

PREPARATION TIME 10 minutes
COOKING TIME 15–20 minutes
SERVES 4–6

1 Drop the chestnuts into a food processor and finely chop (or do it by hand).
2 Mix with the remaining ingredients, adding enough cream to bind the mixture. Use to stuff the neck end of the bird. (Never put stuffing in the body cavity as it prevents air from circulating and therefore the bird from cooking. Also, the stuffing may be undercooked.) Alternatively, for stuffing balls, roll the stuffing into 12–15 walnut-sized (2.5cm/1in) balls. Place on a lightly greased baking tray and roast in the oven for 15–20 minutes, turning once during cooking.

WATCH OUT FOR chestnuts. Most people with a nut allergy can eat them, but if in any doubt, see the variation below.

VARIATIONS Chestnuts can be easily replaced with the same quantity of dried apricots or a mix of dried apricots and prunes.
  You can also make this stuffing without sausage meat by doubling the amount of chestnuts and breadcrumbs. This version is best used to stuff the bird rather than as stuffing balls.

 ### dairy free
also egg & nut free

Follow the recipe on the left, but substitute dairy-free spread for the butter and use soya cream alternative in place of the cream.

 ### gluten free
also egg & nut free

Follow the recipe on the left, but substitute stale (or lightly toasted) gluten-free breadcrumbs for the ordinary ones. If using with sausage meat, make sure the sausage is gluten-free, too. Please note that this version makes a smaller quantity than the others as gluten-free bread is denser.

◀ Pictured on pages 112–113

TIP I use cooked chestnuts – either vacuum-packed or canned – for this recipe, but you could cook your own. To do so, you'll need about 450g (1lb) of chestnuts. Slit the skin on one side of each chestnut and boil in water until tender for about 20 minutes. Leave in the pan to cool slightly then remove them from the pan, one at a time, and peel off the shell and inner skin.

SAUCES, DRESSINGS & ACCOMPANIMENTS

214

Vegetable gravy

This is for when you'd like some luscious gravy but, until you've roasted or grilled the meat, you haven't any juices to make it with. If you don't want a last-minute rush, make some in advance. The browned vegetables and seasonings provide colour and flavour, and it's free of all the "Big Four" allergens and vegetarian-friendly, too.

    dairy, egg, gluten & nut free

1 tbsp flavourless nut-free
  vegetable oil
1 onion, chopped
1 carrot, chopped
1 celery stick, chopped
1 tsp soft dark brown sugar
1 bay leaf
1 tsp mustard powder
1 tsp Worcestershire sauce
450ml (15fl oz) vegetable stock,
  made with vegetable cooking
  water, or plain water

2 tsp vegetable stock powder
1–2 tbsp cornflour
1–2 tbsp water
salt and freshly ground black pepper

PREPARATION TIME 15 minutes
COOKING TIME 18 minutes
SERVES 4

1 Heat the oil in a saucepan. Add the vegetables and fry, stirring, until lightly golden, 3 minutes.
2 Add the sugar and continue to fry the mixture over a moderate heat, stirring all the time, for 5 minutes, until richly browned. Take care not to let it burn.
3 Add the bay leaf, mustard powder, and Worcestershire sauce and stir in the stock or water and stock powder. Bring to the boil, stirring. Reduce the heat and simmer gently until the vegetables are really soft, about 10 minutes.
4 For smooth, glossy gravy, strain the liquid then return it to the rinsed-out saucepan. Blend the cornflour with the water and stir into the liquid (use the smaller quantities for thinner gravy, the larger ones for thicker gravy). Bring to the boil and boil for 1 minute, stirring. Season to taste.

WATCH OUT FOR Worcestershire sauce and mustard powder as they may contain gluten. Make sure you use gluten-free versions, if necessary. Check that your stock is gluten free or dairy free, if need be.

SAUCES, DRESSINGS & ACCOMPANIMENTS

Chantilly topping

Chantilly is cream that has been whipped and sweetened and flavoured with vanilla. Below is a delicious problem-solving version for dairy avoiders to use wherever a recipe calls for whipped cream.

    dairy, egg, gluten and nut free

2 tsp powdered gelatine
5 tsp water
240ml (8fl oz) soya alternative to single cream
2 tbsp icing sugar, sifted
1 tsp vanilla extract

PREPARATION TIME 10 minutes
plus chilling time
MAKES about 300ml (10fl oz)

1 Sprinkle the gelatine over the water in a small heatproof bowl. Leave to soften for 5 minutes. Stand the bowl in a pan of gently simmering water and stir until dissolved completely.
2 Whip the soya cream in a food mixer or with an electric or hand whisk to incorporate air and thickness.
3 Whisk in the sugar then the gelatine and the vanilla extract and chill for about 40 minutes, until just set. Whisk again just before using to fluff up the topping.
Pictured opposite ▶

VARIATION The standard, dairy-based Chantilly cream is also egg, gluten, and nut free. Whip 240ml (8fl oz) of double or whipping cream. As it starts to thicken, add 1–2 tablespoons of sifted icing sugar and ½ teaspoon of vanilla extract and whisk again to incorporate.

TIP For a vanilla bean-flecked topping, split ¼ of a vanilla pod, scrape the contents into the topping, and mix.

Cashew cream

This is another tasty and useful cream for topping fresh fruit and desserts or to stir into soups for added richness. It is the consistency of thick double cream but is dairy free.

   dairy, egg & gluten free

for the cashew cream
55g (2oz) unsalted cashews
120ml (4fl oz) water
for sweet cashew cream
½ tsp vanilla extract
¼ tsp maple syrup

PREPARATION TIME 5 minutes
MAKES about 175ml (6fl oz)

1 In a food processor blend the cashews and half the water to a thick paste (about 2 minutes), stopping and scraping down the sides as necessary.
2 Slowly add the remaining water through the funnel or top and blend until smooth (about 2 minutes). To make sweet cashew cream, blend in the vanilla extract and maple syrup.

nut free
also dairy, egg & gluten free

It would be impossible to make a nut-free cashew cream. Use ordinary double cream, soya cream alternative, or Chantilly topping (see above).

TIP Thin with a little extra water if a runny cream is required.

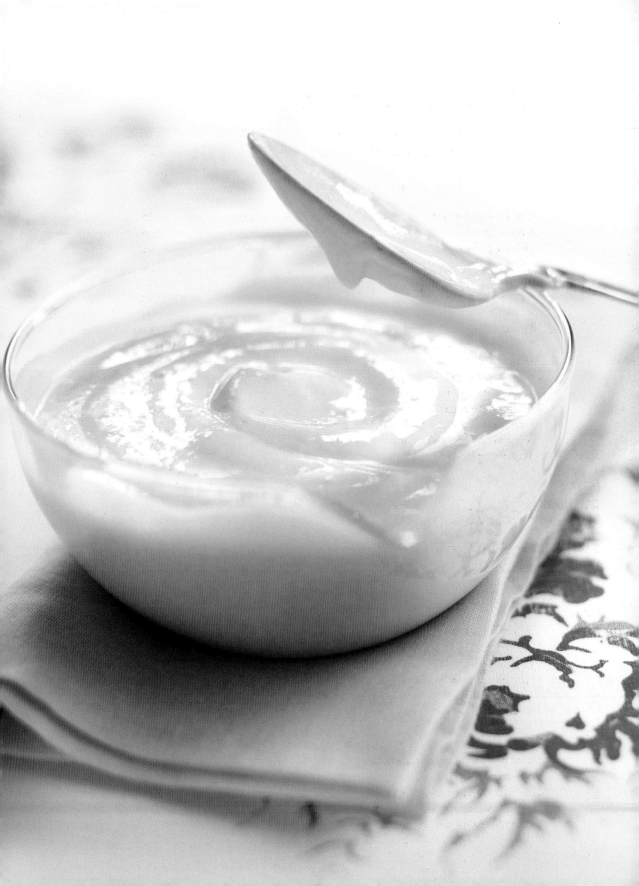

Resources

SUPPORT ORGANIZATIONS

Allergy UK
Helpline: 01322 619 898
info@allergyuk.org
www.allergyuk.org
A national medical charity dealing with allergy, chemical sensitivity, and food intolerance.

Anaphylaxis Campaign
Tel: 01252 546100
Helpline: 01252 542029
www.anaphylaxis.org.uk
Offers support and information and campaigns for people with life-threatening allergic reactions.

British Society for Allergy and Clinical Immunology (BSACI)
Tel: 020 7404 0278
info@bsaci.org
www.bsaci.org
Produces a regularly updated list of NHS allergy clinics throughout the country.

Coeliac UK
Tel: 01494 437278
Helpline: 0870 444 8804
admin@coeliac.co.uk
www.coeliac.co.uk
The UK organization for information and advice for people with coeliac disease.

The Food Allergy and Anaphylaxis Network (FAAN)
www.foodallergy.org
US-based organization dedicated to providing information on all aspects of allergy.

Food Standards Agency
Tel: 020 7276 8000
Publications: 0845 606 0667
www.foodstandards.gov.uk

MedicAlert®
Tel: 020 7833 3034
Helpline: 0800 581420
info@medicalert.org.uk
www.medicalert.org.uk
Wearable emergency identification items for people with hidden medical conditions and allergies. Supported by a 24-hour emergency helpline, which accepts reverse charge calls from anywhere in the world in over 100 languages.

USEFUL FOOD SUPPLIERS

Alprosoya
www.alprosoya.co.uk
Leading manufacturer of soya-based alternatives to milk, cream, yogurt and desserts. Products widely available in supermarkets.

Clearspring
Tel: +44 (0)20 8749 1781
info@clearspring.co.uk
www.clearspring.co.uk
Great for high quality organic and traditional European and Far Eastern foods, many of which are nut, dairy, or gluten free.

Crayves
www.crayves.co.uk
For delicious organic wheat-, gluten- and dairy-free muffins, cereals, and baked goods.

Doves Farm
www.dovesfarm.co.uk
Producers of organic gluten-free flours and mixes, breakfast cereals and cereal bars, savoury biscuits, quick yeast, and flapjacks.

Ecomil
www.ecomil.com
Leading European manufacturer of a wide range of organic non-dairy nut drinks.

Glutafin
Glutafin Careline: 01225 711 801
glutenfree@nutricia.co.uk
www.glutafin.co.uk
Emphasizes enjoyment of eating and cooking, with a wide range of tasty gluten-free products. Good tips on how to make the most of their flour mixes.

Gluten Free Foods
www.glutenfree-foods.co.uk
For gluten-free biscuits, bread, cakes, cereals, crackers and crispbreads, flour and bread mixes, pasta, and savoury snacks.

Goodness Direct
Tel: 0871 871 6611 (office hours or answer phone)
info@GoodnessDirect.co.uk
www.goodnessdirect.co.uk
Great place for specialist diet supplies from xanthan gum to dairy-free cheeses – all home-delivered.

Holland and Barrett
www.hollandandbarrett.com
A UK-wide health food chain

selling mainly grocery and packaged goods. A few branches have refrigerated sections.

Infinity foods
www.infinityfoods.co.uk
For organic products such as gluten-free grains, speciality and gluten-free flours, dried fruit, nuts and seeds, beans, and pulses.

Japanese Kitchen
Tel: +44 (0)20 8788 9014
info@japanesekitchen.co.uk
www.japanesekitchen.co.uk
Brilliant online site for Japanese ingredients including maccha, miso, and nori.

Juvela
www.juvela.co.uk
For gluten-free bread, biscuits, pasta, pizza bases, plus useful information on coeliac disease and on supplies on prescription.

Kallo Foods
www.kallofoods.com
For every kind and flavour of rice cakes plus other snack foods.

Kinnerton Confectionery
www.kinnerton.com
The first confectioner in the world to offer chocolates that are manufactured in a nut-free zone. Has luxury chocolate ranges and cartoon character confectionery.

Lactofree
www.lactofree.co.uk
Real cow's milk with the lactose removed by gentle filtration.

Yoghurt and cheese products are also available.

Marigold Health Foods
www.marigoldhealthfoods.com
Delicious vegetable bouillon powder (including some gluten free) and nutritional yeast flakes (for cheeseless dairy-free sauces).

Orgran
www.orgran.com
Terrific supplier of everything from gluten-free pastas to egg-free pancake mixes. A leading brand to look out for as it's totally focused on health and nutrition.

Plamil Foods
www.plamilfoods.co.uk
Supply egg-free mayonnaise, dairy-free chocolate and carob, and quality alternatives to milk.

Redwood Foods
www.redwoodfoods.co.uk
Dairy-free cheese alternatives that melt, taste, look, and even smell like cheese. Cheezly range now includes "super-melting" Cheddar and Mozzarella-style slices, as well as blocks in Edam, Gouda, and Mozzarella flavours.

Rice Dream
www.tastethedream.eu
A lactose-free milk alternative for anyone who is lactose intolerant or allergic to milk protein.

Sanchi Japanese Foods
www.sanchi.co.uk
Sells tamari – a gluten-free soy

sauce suitable for coeliacs and people who are gluten intolerant.

Suma
www.suma.co.uk
Independent wholesaler and distributor of vegetarian, fairly traded, organic, ethical, and natural products. Good for dairy-free spreads.

Tofutti
www.tofutti.com
Dairy-free products from a US company, some of them available in the UK. Good source of soya cream cheese.

Trufree
www.trufree.co.uk
A useful website with a large range of wheat- and gluten-free products widely available in "free from" sections in supermarkets.

Village Bakery
www.village-bakery.com
Organic, artisanal wheat-free, gluten-free, and dairy-free breads, cakes, bars, and biscuits produced to high standards in a dedicated contamination-free bakery.

BOOKS

Let's Eat Out: Your Passport to Living Gluten and Allergy Free. Kim Koeller and Robert La France. R&R Publishing.
www.allergyfreepassport.com
A good book for coeliacs, with a very useful associated website.

Index

INDEX

Acknowledgments

To my family: allergic Archie, non-allergic Ben and generally intolerant Guy, my mother Lily who is the reason I know how to cook, and my mother-in-law Mollie for taking the trouble to find things that Archie can eat. My thanks to Lucy for being the most intelligent and inquisitive cook I know, to Michelle and Tony for keeping the ship afloat, to the Prof for Italian accents and children's stories, and to the Kit Cat girls for a good time.

I'm grateful to Dr Adam Fox for bringing his medical expertise to this book, to the allergy team at St Mary's Hospital, to Westminster Community Children's Nursing Team, and to Mrs. Hampton and Connaught House School for taking such good care of Archie. I'd like to acknowledge the Anaphylaxis Campaign for their indefatigable work on behalf of people with serious allergies, and, of course, Allergy UK for their support for this book.My thanks also to Professor Lesley Regan for introducing me to the doughty Maggie Pearlstine.

With much gratitude to Mary-Clare Jerram for commissioning this book, to Esther Ripley for editing it with calm and grace, to all the team at DK, in particular Penny Warren, Marianne Markham, Anne Fisher, Vicky Read, and Helen Murray, and to Carolyn Humphries, in appreciation of the knowledge and skills she has brought to bear on this project. Finally, a great deal of credit is due to the team who made the photographs and food in this book look so beautiful; my thanks to art director Luis Peral, photographer Kate Whitaker, prop stylist Chloe Brown, and food stylist Sarah Tildesley.

Alice Sherwood

Alice Sherwood is a writer and multimedia producer whose son has serious nut and egg allergies. She lives in London and spends holidays on the family farm in Wales where her cooking is inspired by the delicious local produce.

Unhappy with the range of existing recipe books for allergy sufferers, which mostly offered unappetizing concoctions, Alice decided to create her own. She is fascinated by the challenge of using different ingredients without compromising at all on taste, her degree in chemistry helping her find the best ways of compensating for the way gluten in flour, for example, gives bread its texture. This book is the result of her years of searching for, devising, and testing recipes that her whole family could enjoy and that fit in with her busy lifestyle.

Publisher's acknowledgments

Dorling Kindersley would like to thank Carolyn Humphries for testing the recipes and giving invaluable advice; Chloe Brown for prop styling; Sue Bosanko for the index; Katie Hardwicke for proofreading; Angela Baynham and Zia Allaway for editorial assistance; and Jack Fisher and Stevie Hope for being our models (p.27).

Picture credits:

The publisher would like to thank the following for their kind permission to reproduce their photographs: Corbis: 28, and 15 (used on tint boxes throughout Chapter 1).